Ion Channels and Genetic Diseases

Society of General Physiologists Series • Volume 50

Ion Channels and Genetic Diseases

Society of General Physiologists • 48th Annual Symposium

Edited by
David C. Dawson
Department of Physiology, University of Michigan, Ann Arbor, Michigan
and
Raymond A. Frizzell
Department of Cell Biology and Physiology, University of Pittsburgh School of Medicine, Pittsburgh, Pennsylvania

Marine Biological Laboratory
Woods Hole, Massachusetts

7–11 September 1994

New York

Library of Congress Catalog Card Number 95-067143
ISBN 0-87470-057-4
Printed in the United States of America

Contents

Preface

This volume is a collection of invited contributions from the 48th Annual Symposium of the Society of General Physiologists, Ion Channels and Genetic Diseases. The Symposium, held September 7–11, 1994, at the Marine Biological Laboratory in Woods Hole, Massachusetts, brought together scientists representing the broad spectrum of disciplines that have converged to produce our current understanding of the role of ion channel gene mutations in inherited disorders. The articles present the problem of channel-related diseases from the varied perspectives of molecular genetics, ion channel biophysics, molecular biology, and integrative physiology. The contributions included here cover the identification of disease-related genes, the effect of mutations on protein structure and function, the impact of channel dysfunction on the cell and organ physiology and the development of therapeutic strategies for overcoming the consequences of inherited defects.

The Symposium was aptly subtitled by our keynote speaker, Francis Collins, as "Worlds in Collusion," a reference to the fact that the discovery of single gene diseases that are caused by dysfunctional ion channels has produced an exciting interface where basic science and medicine meet in a way that enhances both disciplines. The understanding of the molecular basis of disease has been advanced rapidly by the use of high-resolution electrophysiological techniques to probe the functional properties of mutant ion channels. In turn, the existence of inherited channel disorders has been the key to the identification of genes encoding ion channels that had been inferred previously only on the basis of their function. This exciting interchange was highlighted by a session on "Late-breaking Science" that featured seven short presentations of new findings related to genes of clinical interest. And rapid progress continues. At the meeting in September 1994, Mark Keating (page 53) described the search for genes that underly the Long QT Syndrome. Five months later, in the March 10, 1995 issue of *Cell,* he and his colleagues reported the identification of two ion channel genes that are mutated in this disease.

The symposium was entirely supported by contributions from Foundations and the Biotechnology Industry. A lead gift from the Cystic Fibrosis Foundation early in the planning phase catalyzed our fund-raising efforts. We also received grants from the Muscular Dystrophy Association and the March of Dimes Birth Defects Foundation. We are grateful for generous contributions from Amgen, Inc., Axon Instruments, Inc., Merck, Miles, Inc., Pfizer, Inc., SmithKline Beecham, The Upjohn Company, and Warner Lambert-Parke Davis. The broad base of support for this conference underlines the scientific excitement generated by the collusion of genetics and ion channel physiology and the potential importance of the research represented here for future therapies.

We are particularly grateful to Jane Leighton and Susan Judd for their expert management of the Symposium and to John Burris and the Marine Biological Laboratory for their hospitality. The project would not have been possible without the assistance of Myrna Pancost in Ann Arbor and Jan Tidwell in Birmingham.

Chapter 1

Models of Protein Structure

Structural Models of Na^+, Ca^{2+}, and K^+ Channels

H. Robert Guy and Stewart R. Durell

Laboratory of Mathematical Biology, DCBDC, National Cancer Institute, National Institutes of Health, Bethesda, Maryland 20892

The most serious impediment in the field of ion channel research is the lack of detailed, experimentally determined structural models. These structures are vital for understanding how channels function, how drugs and toxins modulate these functions, and how naturally occurring genetic mutations lead to disease. Unfortunately, the very nature of membrane-bound ion channel proteins makes them extremely difficult to study by crystallographic and NMR methods. As a confounding factor, funding agencies have been reluctant to sponsor these long-term structure determination projects, which admittedly have uncertain futures.

In light of these problems, a large multidisciplinary effort has arisen to determine structural information about ion channels using more accessible, albeit less certain methods. Our contribution to this process has been to combine the available experimental data with structure prediction principles to develop molecular models of the ion channel proteins. This is an iterative procedure, where the models are used to suggest further experiments, and the resulting data are used to refine the models. For example, mutagenesis experiments have been very effective in verifying many features of the early voltage-gated channel models, such as which sequence segments span the membrane and form the voltage sensor, inactivation gate, selectivity filter, and ligand binding sites (Guy and Durell, 1994). Likewise, results of mutagenesis experiments have been instrumental in developing our latest refinements of the outer vestibules and ion-selective portions of K^+, Na^+, and Ca^{2+} channels. Here we present these latest models and new models of the entire transmembrane and outer portions of the inward-rectifying, ROMK1 channels.

Na^+ and Ca^{2+} Channel Outer Vestibules and Ion-selective Regions

The mutagenesis experiments described below have confirmed our prediction that the P segments (also called SS1 and SS2 in Na^+ channels and H5 in K^+ channels) form the inner pore and ion-selective filter of K^+, Na^+, and Ca^{2+} channels. In our first models of Na^+ channels (Guy and Seetharamulu, 1986), we suggested that the P segments of repeats I to III each form a short α-helical hairpin, and that the negatively charged faces of the second helix form the ion-selective lining of the pore. Since then we have considered many other possibilities: e.g., a helix followed by a β strand (Guy, 1990; Guy and Conti, 1990), a β hairpin that assembles into a β barrel (Durell and Guy, 1992), and a helix followed by a random coiled structure in K^+ channels (Guy and Durell, 1993). Recent analysis of the expanded set of P segment sequences and new experimental data from Na^+ and Ca^{2+} channels have lead us to return to the original helical hairpin motif. However, now the ion-selective region and tetrodotoxin (TTX) and saxitoxin (STX) binding site is postulated to be formed by the central residues that link the two helices and/or by the residues that initiate the second helix. In addition, the helices are no longer postulated to be oriented parallel to the pore's axis, but rather are tilted so that they form a cone-shaped outer vestibule.

A representation of P segment sequences is shown in Fig. 1. To simplify the comparison of homologous sequences, the numbers have been adjusted to match the aligned prolines of the K$^+$ channels and of repeats II and IV of the Ca^{2+} channels. In the Ca^{2+} channel sequences, the best conserved residues among the four repeats are the threonine at position 12p (T12p), the glutamic acid at position 14p (E14p), and the tryptophan at position 16p (W16p). It is therefore not surprising that mutagenesis experiments have identified the residues at position 14p to be a primary determinant of the ion selectivity. In particular, mutation of the positively charged K14p of repeat III and the uncharged A14p of repeat IV in Na$^+$ channels to negatively charged glutamic acid makes the pore properties resemble those of the

```
                 1p  5p  10p       15p  20p
Na I       FDTFswAFLaLFRlMT----qDfWEnLyqlT
Na II      mhdFfhSFLiVFRVLc----GEwiETmwDcM
Na III     FDNVGlgyLSLLQVAT----FkGWmDIMYAA
Na IV      FeTFGnSMIcLFQitT----saGWdgLLapi
Ca I       FDNFGfSMLtVyQCiT----mEGWtDVLYwv
Ca II      FDNFPQALISVFQVLT----GEdWnsVMYng
Ca III     FDNVlSAMmSLFTVsT----FEGWPqLLYrA
CA IV      FqTFPQAVLLLFRCAT----GEaWqEILLAc
cGMP       ARkYVySLYWStlTLTTi--GEtpPpVrDse
K AKT1     wmrYVTSMYWSITTLTTVGYGDlhPVnTkEM
K EAG      ksmYVTALYFtMTCMTsVGfGnVaAETdnEK
K Shak     FkSiPdAFwWavVTMTTVGYGDmtPVgfwGK
K mSlo     AlTYwecVYLLMVTMSTVGYGDVyAkTTLGR
K Eco      pRSlmTAFYFSIETMSTVGYGDivPVsesAR
K ROMK1     ingmtSAFLFSLETqvTIGYGfrfvTeqcAT
                 1p  5p  10p  15p  20p  25p
```

Figure 1. Sequences of P segments from a Na$^+$ rat brain channel (Noda et al., 1986), a skeletal muscle Ca^{2+} channel (Tanabe, Takeshima, Mikami, Flockerzi, Takahashi, Kangawa, Kojoma, Matsuo, Hirose, and Numa, 1987), a cyclic nucleotide-gated channel (cGMP) (Kaupp, Nidome, Tanabe, Terada, Bonigk, Stühmer, Cook, Kangawa, Matsuo, Hirose, Miyata, and Numa, 1989), KAT1 *Arabidose* K$^+$ channel (Anderson, Huprikar, Kochian, Lucas, and Gaber, 1992), EAG K$^+$ channel (Warmke, Drysdale, and Ganetzky, 1991), *Shaker* voltage-gated K$^+$ channel (Tempel, Papazian, Schwarz, Jan, and Jan, 1987), mSlo Ca^{2+}-activated K$^+$ channel (Butler et al., 1993), a putative K$^+$ channel from *E. coli* (Milkman and McKane-Bridges, 1993), and an inward-rectifying K$^+$ channel, ROMK1 (Ho, Nichols, Lederer, Lytton, Vassilev, Kanazirska, and Herbert, 1993). Na$^+$ and Ca^{2+} channel segments are numbered beginning with the first proline in the repeats II and IV of Ca^{2+} channels (*top*) and K$^+$ channel segments beginning with the first proline in *Shaker* P segment (*bottom*). Residues that occur in three or more sequences in this alignment are bold, those that occur in two sequences are in normal upper case, and those that occur in only one sequence are in lower case. Alignment of Na$^+$ and Ca^{2+} with K$^+$ channels is difficult and ambiguous.

native Ca^{2+} channels (Heinemann, Terlau, and Imoto, 1992*a*). That is, the permeability of the mutant channels to Na$^+$ is blocked by low concentrations of Ca^{2+}, and at higher concentrations the channels become permeant to Ca^{2+}. Likewise, mutating any of the E14p's of Ca^{2+} channels to lysine makes the pore properties similar to those of Na$^+$ channels (Kim, Morii, Sun, Imoto, and Mori, 1993; Mikala, Bahinski, Yatani, Tang, and Schwartz, 1993; Yang, Ellinor, Sather, Zhang, and Tsien, 1993). However, the exact effect of mutating the E14p's of Ca^{2+} channels to lysine or glutamine depends upon which repeat is altered. Thus, in spite of the sequence similarity of the four repeats, the pore is functionally asymmetric. In addition to this, other experiments have shown that calcium channels appear to have two Ca^{2+} binding sites near the extracellular surface (Almers and McCleskey, 1984; Hess and Tsien, 1984). To explain these results, Yang et al. (1993) suggested that some of the

14p glutamic acids form one Ca^{2+} binding site near the extracellular entrance of the pore and others form an additional site farther down inside the pore. In our calcium channel models, the asymmetry and multiple binding sites were approached by considering the differences in the central residues which link the helices of the P segment hairpins (see Fig. 1). For example, glycines occur at position 13p in repeats II and IV and at position 15p in repeats I and III. Due to their enhanced flexibility, glycine residues occur most commonly in the coil and turn segments of proteins (Chou and Fasman, 1978). In addition, highly conserved gylcines tend to be involved in backbone folds that can not be accommodated by the other, more conformationally restricted residue types (Overington, Donnelly, Johnson, Sali, and Blundell, 1992). In the P segment model, repeats II and IV have only two residues, T12p and G13p, linking the helices; whereas, repeats I and III have four nonhelical residues, 12p through 15p, linking the helices (see Fig. 2 *A*). In repeats I and III, residues 13p-16p are postulated to form a type II β turn. This corresponds with the position of the glycines in these repeats, which usually are at the third position of a type II β-turn (Rose, Gierasch, and Smith, 1985). A longer linking segment is also suggested in repeat III by the presence of the proline at position 17p, which is the second residue of the second helix in the model. Due to their unusual structure, proline residues inhibit helical formation in the residues preceding them, but often initiate helices in the residues that follow them (Chou and Fasman, 1978).

As shown in Fig. 2 *B*, the four P segment hairpin structures are assembled, with an approximate fourfold symmetry, about the axis of pore to form a cone-shaped outer vestibule. This model was also designed so that the residues which would be exposed to water in the vestibule are primarily hydrophilic, and the residues which are buried between the helices and the other transmembrane segments are hydrophobic. For the reasons described above, the negatively charged E14p carboxylate groups are made to form the selectivity filter, by being placed at the narrowest portions of the pore. E14p of repeats II and IV form a Ca^{2+} binding site near the extracellular entrance of the pore, and the El4p of repeats I and III form a second site farther down in the pore. In addition to differences in the backbone structure, side chain differences introduce additional asymmetry; e.g., in this model, Ca^{2+} may bind off the pore's axis to D17p of repeat I and E17p of repeat IV in the outer entrance of the selectivity filter and to D15p of repeat II in the inner entrance.

Unfortunately, the P segments of the Na^+ channel are more difficult to model because their sequences differ more among the four repeats than they do for the Ca^{2+} channels. Thus, backbone conformations of the P segment from different repeats are likely to differ even more than in Ca^{2+} channels. Fortunately, however, more experimental data are available for Na^+ channels than for Ca^{2+} channels. For example, not only have mutagenesis experiments indicated that the 14p residues of Na^+ channels are crucial for ion selectivity (described above), but that the binding of TTX and STX depends strongly upon the identity of the 14p and 17p residues in all four repeats (Terlau, Heinemann, Stühmer, Pusch, Conti, Imoto, and Numa, 1991). Conversely, mutation of the residues at positions 9p, 13p, 16p, and 18p appear to have little effect on the binding of these toxins. Also, mutation of the F15p residue of repeat I to cysteine causes a decreased sensitivity to TTX and STX and an increased sensitivity to blockade by zinc (Backx, Yue, Lawrence, Marban, and Tomaselli, 1992; Heineman, Terlau, Stühmer, Imoto, and Numa, 1992*b*; Satin, Kyle, Chen, Bell,

Cribbs, Fozzard, and Rogart, 1992). In contrast, mutation of this residue to tyrosine has little effect.

Fig. 2 *D* displays one of several helical hairpin models we developed for the binding of TTX in Na^+ channels. In accordance with the data described above, each model satisfies the criterion of having almost all of the polar atoms of the toxin

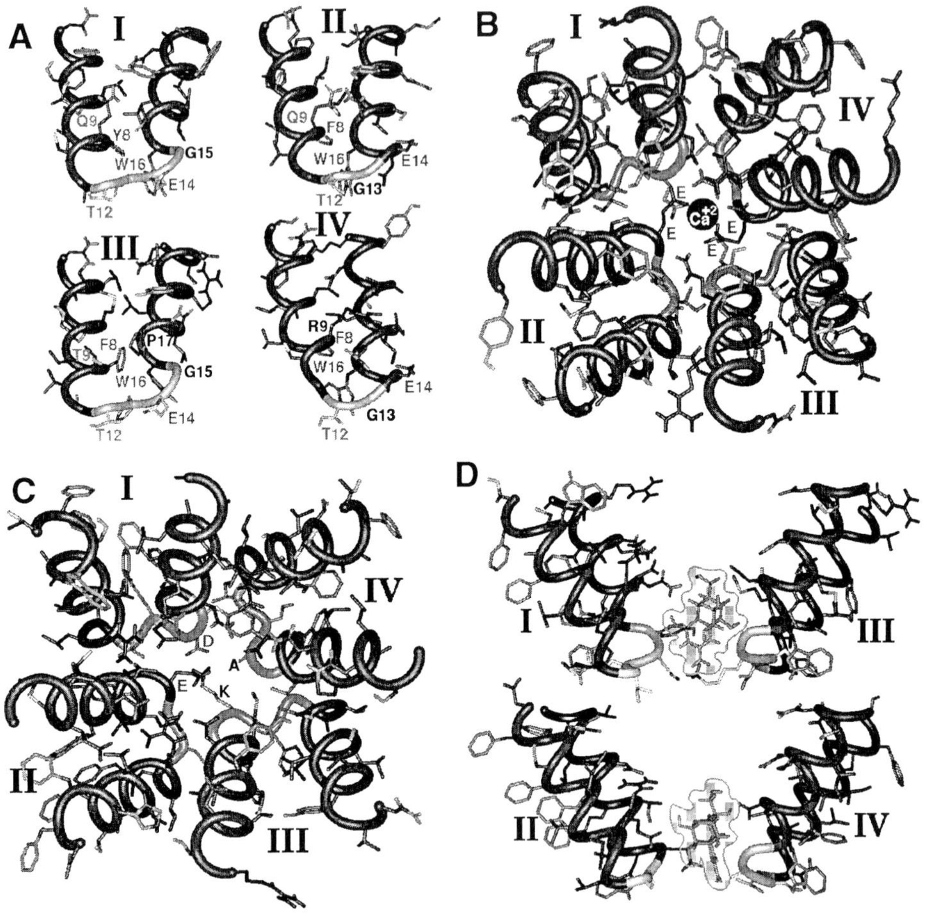

Figure 2. Models of Ca^{2+} and Na^+ channel P segments. (*A*) Models of the four putative P segment helical hairpins of a Ca^{2+} channel viewed as from inside the channel. Top is extracellular. Lightly shaded portions are the putative nonhelical linking regions. (*B*) Model of the four Ca^{2+} channel P segments as assembled in the pore viewed from outside the cell. (*C*) Model of the four P segments of Na^+ channel P segments viewed from outside the cell. (*D*). Side view of Na^+ channel P segments with TTX (*outlined molecule*) bound in the outer entrance of the pore.

forming salt bridges or hydrogen bonds with the 14p and 17p residues of the P segments. Unfortunately, the positions of the helices, conformations of the connecting loops and side chains, and even the order of the repeats remains ambiguous in the Na^+ channel model. It should be noted that Lipkind and Fozzard (1994) proposed an alternate model for the P segments where β hairpins are used instead of helical hairpins. However, the models agree in the sequence location of the turn segments, which are likely the ion-selective region.

K^+ Channel Outer Vestibules and Ion-selective Regions

The K^+ channels are easier to model than the Na^+ and Ca^{2+} channels because they are comprised of four identical subunits rather than four homologous repeats. Thus, it is more reasonable to assume that the channel has fourfold symmetry with respect to the pore's axis, which in turn reduces the number of possible conformations. In addition, there is considerably more mutagenesis data for the K^+ channels than for the other types of channels. However, modeling of the K^+ channel P segments is complicated by the recent findings of Heginbotham, Lu, Abramson, and MacKinnon (1994) which suggest that the ion selective region is not formed by any particular residue side chain, but rather by the polar atoms of the backbone. This also complicates using substitution-type mutagenesis experiments, which just switch side chain identities, for determining which particular residues are involved in ion selectivity. Assuming a hairpin motif, another complicating factor is that the segment of linker residues is substantially longer for the K^+ channels than for the Na^+ or Ca^{2+} channels (see Fig. 1). Finally, the highly conserved glycines at position 15p and 17p in the putative ion selective linker region are more difficult to model because they have considerably more conformational freedom than the other types of residues. However, it will be shown in the following sections how these seeming difficulties may actually provide clues to the structure of the channel.

Due to the ambiguities, we have developed a number of different models for the P segment structure of K^+ channels. Despite the differences, they all share the following attributes, most of which have been predicted by mutagenesis and/or drug-binding experiments. These are (*a*) the 1p to 9p segment forms an α helix that is oriented such that residues 2p and 9p, which have been identified with tetraethylammonium (TEA) binding from the outside (see below), are accessible from the extracellular surface; (*b*) residue 20p, which is on the other end of the P segment, also forms part of the extracellular TEA binding site; (*c*) the backbone carbonyls of the highly conserved G15p-Y16p-G17p segment forms at least part of the ion-selective portion of the pore; (*d*) residues 11p, 12p and 14p, in the middle of the P segment, form at least part of the intracellular TEA binding site; and (*e*) the D18p residue of voltage- and calcium-gated K^+ channels interacts with positively charged residues of charybdotoxin (CTX) when it is bound in the pore. The major differences among the models are in the conformation of the 10p to 20p region in the middle of the P segment sequence. In particular, the models of the pore structure have included four-stranded β barrels (spiraling right, left and straight up and down), short eight-stranded β barrels (formed from the linkers in β-hairpin conformations), a series of vertical β turns, and an extended structure in which the backbone has either a β-strand conformation or a conformation in which the backbone angles of the residues alternate between the values for right- and left-handed α helices (with the conserved 15p and 17p glycine residues assuming the left-handed conformation). We tentatively favor these extended models because they satisfy the experimentally determined criteria described below of having numerous K^+ binding sites and a substantial distance between the intracellular and extracellular TEA binding sites and because they provide a role for the highly conserved glycine residues. The secondary structure predictions of the first α helix and the random coil for the central region are supported by circular dichroism analysis of the isolated *Shaker* P segment in apolar solvent (Peled and Shai, 1993).

Sequence homology and mutagenesis data. Identification of which residues and regions of the sequence are conserved among different protein species is often useful in prediction of protein structure (see Guy and Durell, 1994). Conserved residues generally play important structural and/or functional roles in the protein. Elucidation of these roles is facilitated by correlating the conservation of known functional properties of different proteins with the conservation of the sequences. Fortunately for modeling efforts, there has been a rapid growth in the acquisition of K^+ channel sequences from a variety of families. These families include, voltage-gated, Ca^{2+}-activated, *Eag*, plant, bacterial, and Mg^{2+}-blocked inward-rectifying channels. Because all of the K^+ channels are by definition selective for K^+, comparison of the most distantly related sequences is useful for identifying which residues are essential for K^+ selectivity. For example, 9p-18p is by far the best conserved segment among the distantly related K^+ channel sequences. Within this segment, the Mg^{2+}-blocked inward-rectifying channels (ROMK1, IRKI, GIRK1, KATP) have only five residues (T10p, T13p, G15p, Y16p, and G17p) that are identical to those of most other K^+ channels (see Fig. 1). In addition, many of the residue substitutions are nonconservative; For example, the hydrophobic V9p, M11p, and M19p or V19p residues in the *Shaker* and *Slow-poke* sequences are replaced by the hydrophilic E9p, Q11p, and R19p residues in the ROMK1 sequence, and the negatively charged D18p residue in the *Shaker* and *Slow-poke* sequences is replaced by the hydrophobic F18p residue in the ROMK1 sequence. Of the five conserved residues just described, the two threonine residues are also found conserved in the sequences of the cyclic nucleotide-gated channels (see Fig. 1). Because the cyclic nucleotide-gated channels are nonselective among cations, these threonines are probably conserved for reasons unrelated to K^+ selectivity. Also, T10p, T13p, and Y16p are replaced by S10p, C13p, and F16p in the *Eag* K^+ channel sequence, which leaves the two glycines as the only residues conserved among all of the K^+ channel sequences. This suggests that these glycine residues are crucial for the K^+ selectivity of the channels.

The importance of the two conserved glycines for K^+ selectivity is also indicated by the mutagenesis experiments of Heginbotham et al. (1994), in which every position of the central region of the *Shaker* P segment was mutated one residue at a time. It was found that every residue other than G15p and G17p can be substituted without substantially altering the channels selectivity for K^+ over Na^+. Substitution of either glycine, however, greatly reduces the channel's selectivity among cations. Similarly, Heginbotham, Abramson, and MacKinnon (1992) were able to reproduce the nonselective properties of the cyclic nucleotide-gated channels by deleting the G15p and Y16p residues in the *Shaker* P segment, which is the same as the natural deletion between the two channel sequences (see Fig. 1). In particular, the mutated channel was permeant to both Na^+ and K^+ and was blocked by relatively low concentrations of Ca^{2+}. Likewise, the additional mutation of the D18p residue to E18p resulted in conduction properties similar to those of Ca^{2+} channels, which naturally have the a glutamic acid residue at this location and also lack the G15p and Y16p residues of K^+ channels (see Fig. 1).

These findings have important implications for the structure of the ion-selective portion of the pore. As described above, the mutagenesis results indicate that the highly conserved 15p and 17p glycine residues are the most influential in determining the K^+ selectivity. (It should also be noted that the hydroxyl group of T10p may also play a role in selectivity [Heginbotham et al., 1994]). Because glycine residues lack side chains, we modeled the selectivity filter, which is taken to be the narrowest portion of the pore and in direct contact with the cations, to be formed by the partial negatively charged carbonyl oxygens of the conserved G15p-Y16p-G17p residue backbones (Heginbotham et al., 1994). In addition, we make the assumption that the glycine residues were probably conserved by evolution because they are able to assume a conformation which is energetically unfavorable for other residue types, which is generally what is observed for the highly conserved gylcine residues in soluble proteins (Overington et al., 1992). For this reason, the ion-selective, central region of the P segment would likely not have a regular α helical or β strand conformation. Instead, our models of the K^+ channels have this region of the P segment forming either a random or extended conformation (see Fig. 3).

Multiple K^+ binding sites. Experimental studies have indicated that Ca^{2+}-activated K^+ channels may possess up to four K^+ binding sites in their pore (Neyton and Miller, 1988). Assuming that the sites are arranged single file, this helps constrain the modeling by requiring a long, narrow pore structure. As shown in Fig. 3, this is accomplished by having the highly conserved, ion-selective region of the P segment in an extended conformation, oriented parallel to the axis of the pore. Two conformational extremes are illustrated. Fig. 3 *E* shows the pore when no ions are present, and thus, the amide groups are free to form interstrand hydrogen bonds. This four-stranded structure is very atypical, in that most β barrels have at least six strands which spiral around the axis in a right-handed fashion. However, the lack of interior side chains due to the one-residue–separated positions of the conserved G15p and G17p residues makes this narrow structure feasible. Fig. 3 *F* shows the other extreme, where the amide groups have rotated by 90° so that the carbonyl oxygens can interact with the ions in the pore. To accomplish this, the torsion angles of the residue backbones alternate along the strand between the values for left- and right-handed α helices. Once again, this is feasible due to the fact that the conserved glycine residues lack side chains and are thus able to assume left-handed helical conformations. The V14p and Y16p residues assume the normal right-handed helical torsion values. This peculiar conformation for the strands allows for all the carbonyl oxygens to point into the pore and form K^+ binding sites. Two basic types of binding sites are imagined: one with the ion in the plane of four carbonyl oxygens, and one with the ion in between two planes of four oxygens each (thus, binding to eight oxygens all together). In these models, the pore's lining is envisioned to be a highly dynamic, polarizable structure whose precise conformation is influenced by the location and number of ions in the pore. The examples illustrated are the narrowest pores that we have modeled. The pore may be made larger by adding additional water modelcules.

TEA binding sites. The prediction of a long, extended pore structure is also supported by the data for TEA binding. Many of the different K^+ channel pores are found to be blocked by TEA at two distinct sites; one accessible from outside the cell and the other from inside the cell. From the voltage dependency of binding, it is found that the TEA molecule need not traverse much, if any, of the transmembrane electric field to reach the extracellular site, and only transverses 20% of the field to reach the intracellular site (Miller, 1991). Although electrostatic repulsion between TEA ions at the two sites has been reported (Newland, Adelman, Tempel, and

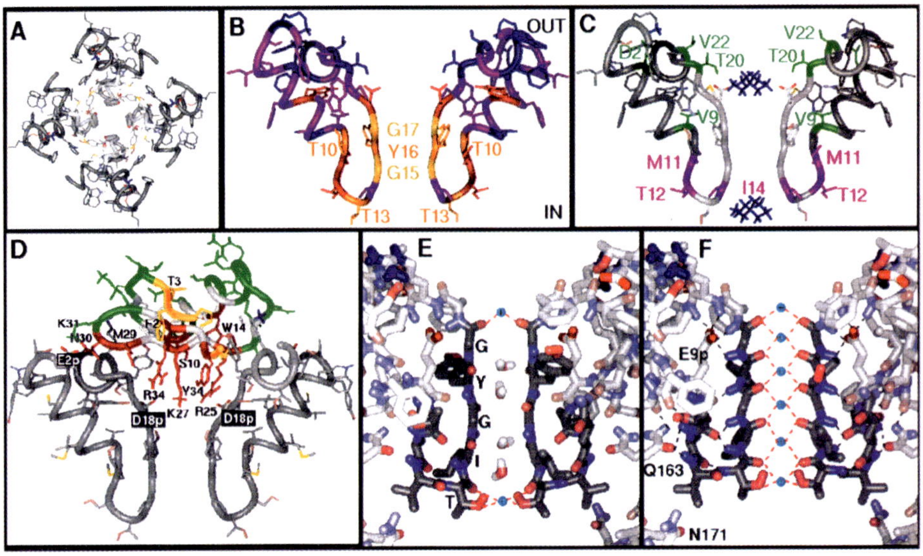

Figure 3. Models of *Shaker* K^+ channel P segments. (*A*) Assembly of four P segments to form outer vestibule and ion-selective region of the channel; view form outside the cell. Dark gray tubes are backbones of α helices; white tubes are random coil backbone. Side chain color code: gray=alkyl carbons, pink=uncharged oxygens, red=negatively charged oxygens, light blue=uncharged nitrogens, yellow=sulfurs. (*B*) Cross-section of outer vestibule and ion-selective region showing two P segments. View is the same as in *A* except monomers are rotated by 90°. Residues are colored coded according to how well they are conserved among distantly related K^+ channels: the number of residue types in all sequences are: yellow=1, orange=2, red=3, purple=4, blue=5. (*C*) Side view of P segments illustrating residues where mutations alter TEA binding from outside (*green*) and inside (*purple*) the cell. TEA molecules (*dark blue*) are ~15 Å apart. (*D*) Illustration of charybdotoxin (CTX) bound in the outer vestibule of a Ca^{2+}-activated mslo channel. CTX residues are colored according to how much mutations affect the off rate of binding: red=large effect, yellow=moderate effect, green=little or no effect. Crucial CTX residues are labeled black and negatively charged channel residues are labeled white. (*E and F*) Side view of putative ion-selective portion of ROMK1 channel in two extreme conformations. In *E*, residues 14p-16p have a β conformation and the pore is filled with water molecules (*pink and white*). In *F*, residues I14p and Y16p have a right handed α type conformation, G15p and G17p have a left handed α type conformation and the pore is filled with K^+ ions (*cyan*). The actual pore is envisioned to be a highly dynamic structure that exists between these extremes most of the time. Q163 and N171 are residues on M2. All backbone atoms are shown. Color code: black=carbons of 10p-17p, white=carbons of other segments, pink=uncharged oxygens of backbone or side chain, red=negatively charged side chain oxygens, light blue=uncharged nitrogens, cyan=potassium ions, red dashed lines=salt bridges, black dashed lines=hydrogen bonds.

Almers, 1992), the fact that they are separated by 80% of the transmembrane electric field indicates a considerable separation distance.

Fig. 3 *C* shows the positions of residues in our model where mutations alter TEA binding at the extracellular (MacKinnon and Yellen, 1990; De Biasi, Kirsch, Drewe, Hartmann, and Brown, 1993) and intracellular (Yellen, Jurman, Abramson, and MacKinnon, 1991; Hartmann, Kirsch, Drewe, Taglialatela, Joho, and Brown, 1991; Choi, Mossman, Aubie, and Yellen, 1993) sites. The 20p residues from the four subunits were positioned near the extracellular entrance to the pore so that when they are tyrosines or phenylalanines their aromatic groups form much of the TEA binding site, as suggested by Heginbotham and MacKinnon (1992). As described above, the extended structure of the pore maximizes the distance between the 14p and 20p residues, which are known to affect intracellular and extracellular TEA binding, respectively. The experimental data for the mutation of the 9p residue to histidine (De Biasi et al., 1993) is especially interesting because it alters the effects of extracellular TEA, zinc, histidine reagents, and changes in pH even though it is close in sequence to the M11p and T12p residues, where mutations affect the binding of intracellular TEA. In the models, the 9p residue, which is a valine in the *Shaker* and *Slow-poke* sequences, is buried in the nonpolar interior of the protein near the extracellular entrance to the pore. In the inward rectifier (ROMK1) the 9p residue is a buried glutamic acid; however, it is able to form neutralizing hydrogen bonds with the amide groups of four proximal residues in the model (see Fig. 3 *F*). Although the 9p residue is not directly in the pore lining or TEA binding site, as suggested by DeBiasi et al. (1993), it is in a crucial position such that the nonconservative mutation to histidine could easily affect the pore's structure and properties, as described above. The possibility that this mutation alters the backbone conformation of the channel is suggested by the finding that the mutation of the 9p residue to histidine also effects the channel's activation gating kinetics (De Biasi et al., 1993). Mutagenesis experiments also indicate that 2p is sufficiently near the extracellular TEA binding site to affect TEA binding by an indirect electrostatic mechanism (MacKinnon and Yellen, 1990). In analogy to the Na^+ and Ca^{2+} channel models, we have modeled the K+ channel 1p-10p segment as an α helix. This model has the advantage of placing 2p and 9p relatively near each other on the face of the helix that is postulated to form part of the lining of the outer vestibule.

CTX binding. Docking of a charybdotoxin (CTX) molecule into the outer vestibule model was used to constrain the orientations of the helical portions of the P segments that are postulated to form the outer vestibule of the channel models. CTX is a scorpion toxin peptide that is known to block the extracellular entrance of some voltage-gated and Ca^{2+}-activated K^+ channels (Anderson, MacKinnon, Smith, and Miller, 1988; MacKinnon and Miller, 1988). Fortunately, the three-dimensional structure of the peptide in solution has been determined by NMR (Bontems, Gilquin, Roumestand, Menez, and Toma, 1992). Mutation of the positively charged K27 of CTX to a neutral residue has been shown to reduce the overall binding affinity and eliminate the ability of extracellular CTX to compete with intracellular K^+ (Park and Miller, 1992). This strongly suggests that the positively charged ammonium group of K27 normally reaches into one of the K^+ binding sites in the ion-selective region of the pore. As depicted in Fig. 3 *D*, the K27 CTX side chain is positioned inside the ring of the four negatively charged D18p residues of the P segments. This orientation for the CTX molecule is also supported by the finding that mutation of the S10, W14, R25, M29, N30, R34, and Y36 residues, which are on the same face of the CTX molecule as K27, significantly affect the dissociation rate from Ca^{2+}-activated K^+ channels. Likewise, nonconservative mutations of residues on the opposite side of the CTX molecule have little effect on the dissociation rate (Stampe, Kolmakova-Partensky, and Miller, 1994). In the model shown in Fig. 3 *D*, the positively charged R25 and R34 residues of CTX join with the K27 residue to form salt bridges with the four D18p residues. In addition, the K11 and K31 residues of

CTX form salt bridges with the E2p residues of adjacent subunits on the periphery of the outer vestibule. This interaction is supported by the finding that in the *Shaker* channel the mutation of D2p to asparagine eliminates the binding of CTX (MacKinnon and Yellen, 1990). Also in the model, the aromatic F2 and W14 residues of CTX bind at the beginning of the second helix of opposite subunits and interact with the Y20p and K22p residues of the P segments. Aromatic residues are known to have favorable interactions with other aromatics (Burley and Petsko, 1985) and with positively charged residues in known protein structures. Thus, CTX can dock into the model of the outer vestibule in a manner in which the interactions between the toxin and pore are highly complementary and consistent with the experimental findings.

Inward Rectifying K^+ Channels

A major shortcoming of the models described so far is that they lack the surrounding transmembrane segments (S1–S6), which would likely influence the predicted conformations of the P segments. Although we have attempted to make atomic-scale models for the surrounding segments of voltage-gated (Durell and Guy, 1992) and Ca^{2+}-activated K^+ channels, the structures are too large to predict with much certainty. However, the situation is simplified for the inward-rectifying and homologous K^+ channel proteins, which probably have only two transmembrane helices (M1 and M2) per subunit in addition to the P segments.

Fig. 4 displays the model of the M1, M2, extracellular linkers and P segments of the ROMK1 channel. The procedures used to build the models has been described previously (Durell and Guy, 1992). In developing these models, we attempt to optimize the following interactions:

(*a*) Side chain-water interactions. Polar residues are made to contact other polar residues or the solvent.

(*b*) Side chain-lipid interactions. Nonpolar residues are either buried in the protein or made to be in contact with the alkyl chains of the membrane.

(*c*) Side chain-side chain interactions. A disulfide bride is formed between C121 and C153. Salt bridges are formed from D108 and E111 to R147, from D116 and E123 to R118, and from E152 to H106. Hydrogen bonds are formed between S130 and E153, Y100 and S135, S135 and S164, and W92 and Q139. A cluster of aromatic side chains is formed by W92, F95, W99, Y100, F134, Y144, F146, and F148 (see Fig. 4, *C* and *E*).

(*d*) Backbone hydrogen bonds. Virtually all backbone polar atoms are required to form hydrogen bonds. Most backbone polar atoms that are within regular secondary structures, i.e., α or 3_{10} helices or β sheets form hydrogen bonds to other backbone atoms. At the ends of helices or in "random coil" segments some of these atoms may hydrogen bond to side chain atoms, e.g., K107 interacts with the COOH terminal of M1, D108 and T139 with the NH_2 terminal of the first P-segment helix, T133, Q139 and Q164 with the COOH terminal of this helix, Q164 to the loop region that follows it, E137 with the pore-lining segment and the NH_2 terminal of the 3_{10} helix postulated to link the lining to M2, and T119 with the NH_2 terminal of a surface helix in the M1-P linking segment (see Fig. 4 *C*). The M1-P linking segment is postulated to have a random coil segment located on the extracellular surface of the protein where some unpaired backbone polar atoms hydrogen bond to water. Within the pore, some backbone oxygens may interact with ions (see Fig. 3 *F*). The putative random coil segments contain proline and glycine residues that tend to disrupt helices and β sheets, whereas the putative helices do not contain these residues except for prolines at some of the NH_2 termnals where they are energetically favorable.

(*e*) Residue packing. The structure is modeled so that the atoms within the protein pack tightly together with no large cavities within the protein (see Fig. 4, *D* and *E*).

(*f*) Torsion angles. Residues are modeled with backbone and side chain torsion angles that occur commonly in known protein structures.

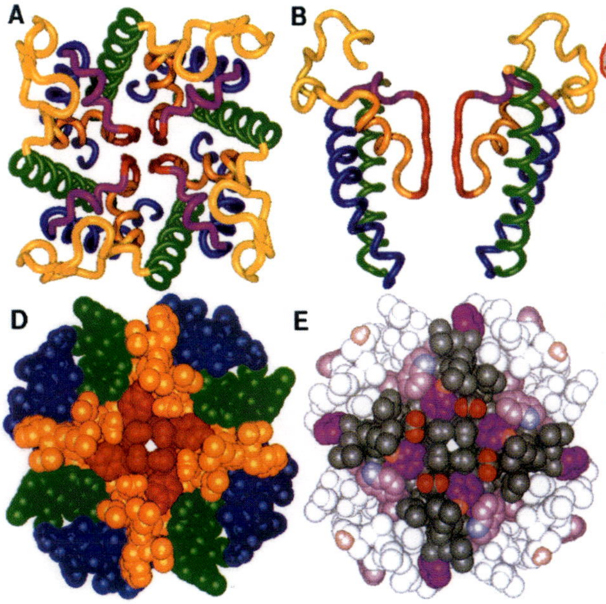

Figure 4. Model of transmembrane and extracellular portions of ROMK1 channel. (*A*) View from outside and (*B*) side view of backbone structure. Segments are color coded as: green = M1, yellow = M1-P extracellular linker, orange = P1, red = P2, purple = P-M2 linker, blue = M2. (*C*) Side view illustrating energetically favorable interactions. Shaded area color code: yellow = disulfide bridge, red = salt bridges, blue = side chain–side chain hydrogen bonds, cyan = side chain–backbone hydrogen bonds, purple = aromatic cluster. Gray backbone = P segment, white backbone = other segments. Polar side chain atoms colored as in Fig. 3 *A*. (*D and E*) Space-filled model of channels cross-section through the P segments illustrating tight packing. (*D*) Colored by segments as in *A* and *B*. (*E*) Colored as in *C* but with aromatic side chain carbon atoms colored purple in P and lavender in other segments. (*F*) Side view illustrating extent of sequence conservation. Yellow residues are identical in all K^+ channel families except *Eag*. Color code for number of residue types in multisequence alignment of inward rectifying K^+ channels: orange = 1, red = 2, purple = 3, blue = 4, gray ≥ 5.

(*g*) Sequence conservation. Special attention is placed on whether a residue is conserved in the family of sequences (Guy and Durell, 1994). As is generally observed for known soluble and transmembrane protein structures, the poorly conserved polar and nonpolar residues are put in contact with either the solvent or the lipid, respectively (see Fig. 4 *F*). In contrast, the conserved residues are used for important structural and/or functional purposes. For example, the putative selectivity filter region is the most highly conserved part of the protein among all K^+ channels. In addition, many of the energetically favorable side chain–side chain and side chain-backbone interactions described above involve residues that are highly conserved within the family of K^+ channels that includes ROMK1.

The most noteworthy aspect of the ROMK1 model is that, beginning with the backbone structure of P segments developed from very distantly related K^+ channels, a model that satisfies all our criteria described above could be made of all the protein segments surrounding the P segment. Although the model of the pore formed by M1 and M2 in the intracellular half of the transmembrane region is more ambiguous, one aspect is consistent with recent experimental findings. N175 has been shown to be involved in the voltage-dependent blockade of ROMK1 by magnesium (Lu and MacKinnon, 1994). This effect has been postulated to be caused by an electrostatic effect. In our models, this residue is on the lining of the pore just beyond the end of the P segment where one might expect magnesium to bind (see Fig. 3 *E*).

Summary

The structure determination of voltage-gated channels by the combination of molecular modeling and mutagenesis experiments is a long term, iterative process. As such, the models should be considered as a work in progress, with changes expected as more data becomes available. The primary role of the models is that they assimilate the known data and provide ideas for further experiments to elucidate the real structures. Although the models presented here have already gone through two or three cycles of development and testing, many aspects remain tentative. Perhaps the most significant result so far is that the P segment was experimentally confirmed to form the ion-selective part of the channel. In a subsequent cycle of testing and modeling, the specific residues responsibility for Na^+ and Ca^{2+} selectivity have been identified and the selectivity filter of K^+ channels is now predicted to be formed not by the side chains, but rather by the carbonyl oxygens of the conserved Gly-Tyr-Gly sequence backbone. As another example, the 9p residue of the P segment of K^+ channels was originally modeled as either being buried in the protein or accessible from inside the cell only. However, once mutation of this residue to histidine was found to affect blockade by extracellular TEA, protons, Zn^{2+} and histidine reagents (DeBiasi et al., 1993), the models were updated to have this and the hydrophilic residues in the first part of P form a helix that comprises part of the extracellular, outer vestibule of the pore. While this motif was used also for Na^+ and Ca^{2+} pore models (see Fig. 2) where the putative helices are amphipathic, it remains to be verified. Modeling of the size and shape of the outer vestibule of K^+ channels was also aided by the data for the binding of CTX in the extracellular entrance to the pore. Similarly, experiments with peptide toxins such as μ and Ω conotoxins may prove useful in modeling the outer vestibules of the Na^+ and/or Ca^{2+} channels.

While important advances have been made, it is important to realize that these approaches are still very new. In the future we are likely to see improvements on both the theoretical and experimental sides which will greatly advance the process. For example, as computational power increases and as methods to calculate protein-ligand interactions improve, it will likely become possible to accurately calculate the binding affinities of toxins such as TTX and STX to the model pore structures of Na^+ and Ca^{2+} channels and compare these with experimental values. This should help discriminate between different pore motifs. Similarly, computational studies of the free energy of ion permeation, such as pursued by Roix and Karplus (1994) and Chiu, Novotny, and Jakobsson (1993), may also greatly assist in understanding the structure of the pore and the mechanisms that enable ion selectivity.

Of course, what we need most is hard structural data; the type obtained by x-ray crystallography, NMR and electron cryomicroscopy. Unfortunately, It is unlikely that high resolution structures of voltage-gated channels will be obtained anytime soon. One reason is that the expression systems needed to produce the necessary quantity of purified protein have only recently been developed (Santacruz-Toloza, Perozo, and Papazian, 1994; Spencer, Takenaka, Aiyar, Ngyen, Grissmer, Gutman, and Chandy, 1994), and many additional difficulties remain to be overcome. However, it may be possible to use synthesized peptide analogues of the P segment with or without other segments to make membrane-bound crystals or water soluble. In this case, structural models will be essential for deciding how to tether the P segments together, and how to make the analogues long enough to span the bilayer or water soluble.

References

Almers, W., and E. W. McCleskey. 1984. Non-selective conductance in calcium channels of frog muscle: calcium selectivity in a single-file pore. *Journal of Physiology.* 353:585–608.

Anderson, C., R. MacKinnon, C. Smith, and C. Miller. 1988. Charybdotoxin block of single Ca^{2+}-activated K^+ channels: effects of channel gating, voltage, and ionic strength. *Journal of General Physiology.* 91:317–333.

Anderson, J. A., S. S. Huprikar, L. V. Kochian, W. J. Lucas, and R. F. Gaber. 1992. Functional expression of a probable *Arabidopsis thaliana* potassium channel in *Saccharomyces cerevisiae. Proceedings of the National Adademy of Sciences, USA.* 89:3736–3740.

Backx, P., D. Yue, J. Lawrence, E. Marban, and G. Tomaselli. 1992. Molecular localization of an ion-binding site within the pore of mammalian sodium channels. *Science.* 257:248–251.

Bontems, F., G. Gilquin, C. Roumestand, A. Menez, and F. Toma. 1992. Analysis of side-chain orgainzation on a refined model of charybdotoxin: structural and functional implications. *Biochemistry.* 31:7756–7764.

Burley, S. K., and G. A. Petsko. 1985. Aromatic–aromatic interaction: a mechanism of protein structure stabilization. *Science.* 229:23–28.

Butler, A., S. Tsunoda, D.P. McCobb, A. Wei, and L. Salkoff. 1993 mSlo, a complex mouse gene encoding 'maxi' calcium-activated potassium channels. *Science.* 261:221–224.

Chiu, S.W., J.A. Novotny, and E. Jakobsson. 1993. The nature of ion and water barrier crossings in a simulated ion channel. *Biophysical Journal.* 64:98–108.

Choi, K. L., C. Mossman, J. Aubie, and G. Yellen. 1993. The internal quaternary ammonium receptor site of *Shaker* potassium channels. *Neuron.* 10:533–541.

Chou, P.Y., and G. D. Fasman. 1978. Empirical predictions of protein conformation. *Annual Review of Biochemistry.* 47:251–276.

De Biasi, M., G. E. Kirsch, J. A. Drewe, H. A. Hartmann, and A. M. Brown. 1993. Cesium selectivity conferred by histidine substitution in the pore of the potassium channel Kv 2.1. *Biophysical Journal.* 64:A341. (Abstr.)

Durell, S. R., and H. R. Guy. 1992. Atomic scale structure and functional models of voltage-gated potassium channels. *Biophysical Journal.* 62:238–250.

Guy, H. R. 1990. Models of voltage- and transmitter-activated channels based on their amino acid sequences. *In* Monovalent Cations in Biological Systems. C. A. Pasternak, editor. CRC Press, Boca Raton, FL. 31–58.

Guy, H. R., and F. Conti. 1990. Pursuing the structure and function of voltage-gated channels. *Trends in Neuroscience.* 13:201–206.

Guy, H. R., and S. R. Durell. 1993. Models of the slowpoke calcium-activated potassium channel. *Biophysical Journal.* 64:A228. (Abstr.)

Guy, H. R., and S. R. Durell. 1994. Using homology in modeling the structure of voltage-gated ion channels. *In* Molecular Evolution of Physiological Processes. D. Fambrough, editor. The Rockefeller University Press, NY. 197–212.

Guy, H. R., and P. Seetharamulu. 1986. Molecular model of the action potential sodium channel. *Proceedings of the National Academy of Sciences, USA.* 83:508–512.

Hartmann, H. A., G. E. Kirsch, J. A. Drewe, M. Taglialatela, R. H. Joho, and A. M. Brown. 1991. Exchange of conduction pathways between two related K^+ channels. *Science.* 251:942–944.

Heginbotham, L., and R. MacKinnon. 1992. The aromatic binding site for tetraethylammonium ion on potassium channels. *Neuron.* 8:483–491.

Heginbotham, L., T. Abramson, and R. MacKinnon. 1992. A functional connection between the pores of distantly related ion channels as revealed by mutant K^+ channels. *Science.* 258:1152–1155.

Heginbotham, L., Z. Lu, T. Abramson, and R. MacKinnon. 1994. Mutations in the K^+ channel signature sequence. *Biophysical Journal.* 66:1061–1067.

Heinemann, S. H., H. Terlau, and K. Imoto. 1992. Molecular basis for pharmacological differences between brain and cardiac sodium channels. *Pflügers Archiv.* 422:90–92.

Heinemann, S. H., H. Terlau, W. Stühmer, K. Imoto, and S. Numa. 1992. Calcium channel characteristics conferred on the sodium channel by single mutations. *Nature.* 356:441–443.

Hess, P., and R. W. Tsien. 1984. Mechanism of ion permeation through calcium channels. *Nature.* 309:453–456.

Ho, K., C. G. Nichols, W. J. Lederer, J. Lytton, P. M. Vassilev, M. V. Kanazirska, and S. C. Hebert. 1993. Cloning and expression of an inwardly rectifying ATP-regulated potassium channel. *Nature.* 262:31–38.

Kaupp, U. B., T. Niidome, T. Tanabe, S. Terada, W. Bonigk, W. Stühmer, N. J. Cook, K. Kangawa, H. Matsuo, T. Hirose, T. Miyata, and S. Numa. 1989. Primary structure and functional expression from complementary DNA of the rod photoreceptor cyclic GMP-gated channel. *Nature.* 342:762–766.

Kim, M.-K., T. Morii, L.-X. Sun, K. Imoto, and Y. Mori. 1993. Structural determinants of ion selectivity in brain calcium channel. *FEBS Letters.* 318:145–148.

Lipkind, G. M., and H. A.Fozzard. 1994. A structural model of the tetrodotoxin and saxitoxin binding site of the Na^+ channel. *Biophysical Journal.* 66:1–13.

Lu, Z., and R. MacKinnon. 1994. Electrostatic tuning of Mg^{2+} affinity in an inward-rectifier K^+ channel. *Nature.* 371:243–246.

Mackinnon, R., and C. Miller. 1988. Mechanism of charybdotoxin block of the high-conductance, Ca^{2+}-activated K^+ channel. *Journal of General Physiology.* 91:335–349.

MacKinnon, R., and G. Yellen. 1990. Mutations affecting TEA blockade and ion permeation in voltage-activated K^+ channels. *Science.* 250:276–279.

Mikala, G., A. Bahinski, A. Yatani, S. Tang, and A. Schwartz. 1994. Differential contribution by conserved glutamate residues to an ion-selectivity site in the L-type Ca^{2+} channel pore. *FEBS Letters.* 335:265–269.

Milkman, R., and M. McKane-Bridges. 1993. An *E. coli* homologue of eukaryotic potassium channels. Genebank entry ECOKCH.

Miller, C. 1991. 1990: Annus mirabilis of potassium channels. *Science.* 252:1092–1096.

Newland, C. F., J. P. Adelman, B. L. Tempel, and W. Almers. 1992. Repulsion between tetraethylammonium ions in cloned voltage-gated potassium channels. *Neuron.* 8:978–982.

Neyton, J., and C. Miller. 1988. Discrete Ba^{2+} block as a probe of ion occupancy and pore structure in the high-conductance Ca^{2+}-activated K^+ channel. *Journal of General Physiology.* 92:569–586.

Noda, M., T. Ikeda, T. Kayano, H. Suzuki, H. Takeshima, M. Kurasaki, H. Takahashi, and S. Numa. 1986. Existence of distinct sodium channel messenger RNAs in rat brain. *Nature.* 320:188–192.

Overington, J., D. Donnelly, M. S. Johnson, A. Sali, and T. L. Blundell. 1992. Environment-specific amino acid substitution tables: tertiary templates and prediction of protein folds. *Protein Science.* 1:216–226.

Park, C. S., and C. Miller. 1992 Interaction of charybdotoxin with permeant ions inside the pore of a K^+ channel. *Neuron.* 9:307–313.

Peled, H., and Y. Shai. 1993 Membrane interaction and self-assembly within phospholipid membranes of synthetic segments corresponding to the H-5 region of the *Shaker* K^+ channel. *Biochemistry.* 32:7879.

Rose, G. D., L. M. Gierasch, and J. A. Smith. 1985. Turns in peptides and proteins. *Advances in Protein Chemistry.* 37:1–109.

Roux, B., and M. Karplus. 1994. Moleucular dynamics simulations of the gramididin channel. *Annual Review Biophysics Biomolecuar Structure.* 23:731–761.

Santacruz-Toloza, L., E. Perozo, and D. M. Papazian. 1994. Purification and reconstitution of functional *Shaker* K channels assayed with a light-driven, voltage-control system. *Biophysical Journal.* 66:A343. (Abstr.)

Satin, J., J. W. Kyle, M. Chen, P. Bell, L. L. Cribbs, H. A. Fozzard, and R. B. Rogart. 1992. A mutant of TTX-resistant cardiac sodium channels with TTX-sensitive properties. *Science* 256:1202–1205.

Spencer. R. H., B. Takenaka, J. Aiyar, A. Ngyen, S. Grissmer, G. A. Gutman, and K. G. Chandy. 1994. Purification and biochemical characterization of a mammalizn K^+ channel protein, Kv1.3. *Biophysical Journal.* 66:A343. (Abstr.)

Stampe, P., L. Kolmakova-Partensky, and C. Miller. 1994. Intimations of K^+ channel structure from a complete functional map of the molecular surface of charybdotoxin. *Biochemistry.* 33:443–450.

Tanabe,T., H. Takeshima, A. Mikami, V. Flockerzi, H. Takahashi, K. Kangawa, M. Kojima, H.

Matsuo, T. Hirose, and S. Numa. 1987. Primary structure of the receptor for calcium channel blockers from skeletal muscle. *Nature.* 328:313–318.

Tempel, B. L., D. M. Papazian, T. L. Schwarz, Y. N. Jan, and L. Y. Jan. 1987. Sequence of a probable potassium channel component encoded at *Shaker* locus of *Drosophila*. *Science.* 237:770–775.

Terlau, H., S. H. Heinemann, W. Stühmer, M. Pusch, F. Conti, H. Imoto, and S. Numa. 1991. Mapping the site of tetrodotoxin and saxitoxin of sodium channel II. *FEBS Letters.* 293:93–96.

Warmke, J., R. Drysdale, and B. Ganetzky. 1991. A distinct potassium channel polypeptide encoded by the *Drosophila eag* locus. *Science.* 252:1560–1562.

Yang, J., P. T. Ellinor, W. A. Sather, J.-F. Zhang, and R. W. Tsien. 1993. Molecular determinants of Ca^{2+} selectivity and ion permeation in L-type Ca^{2+} channels. *Nature* 366:158–161.

Yellen, G., M.E. Jurman, T. Abramson, and R. MacKinnon. 1991. Mutations affecting internal TEA blockade identify the probable pore-forming region of a K^+ channel. *Science.* 251:939–942.

Nucleotide Domains in Transport ATPases: Structure-Function and Relationship to Disease

Philip J. Thomas, Young Hee Ko, Ponniah Shenbagamurthi, and Peter L. Pedersen

Laboratory of Molecular and Cellular Bioenergetics, Department of Biological Chemistry, The Johns Hopkins University, School of Medicine, Baltimore, Maryland 21205-2185

It is known that over 50 transport systems exist which exhibit putative ATP binding domains (Higgins, 1992). Collectively these are referred to as the ABC transporter supergene family. They are referred to also as M-type ATPases (Pedersen and Amzel, 1993) because of their structural similarity to the multidrug resistance protein (MDR-1 or P-glycoprotein), and in other cases as traffic ATPases (Doige and Ferro-Luzzi Ames, 1993). Among this class of transporters are MDR-1, MDR-2, CFTR, TAP 1 and 2, STE6, and over 25 bacterial transporters. Most have two nucleotide domains.

A major effort of this laboratory has been to understand structural-functional relationships within the nucleotide binding domains of transport ATPases. Specifically, the nucleotide binding domains of the CFTR protein (cystic fibrosis transmembrane conductance regulator) and the mitochondrial ATPase/ATP synthase complex (an F-type ATPase) have been extensively studied. To this end, we have overexpressed these domains in *Escherichia coli* (Garboczi, Hullihen, and Pedersen, 1988; Lee, Garboczi, Thomas, and Pedersen, 1990; Ko, Thomas, and Pedersen, 1993), chemically synthesized key regions containing the nucleotide binding consensus sequences (Thomas, Shenbagamurthi, Ysern, and Pedersen, 1991; Ko, Thomas, and Pedersen, 1994), and used both mutational analysis (Garboczi, Thomas, and Pedersen, 1990; Thomas, Garboczi, and Pedersen, 1992*a*) and biophysical approaches (Thomas, Shenbagamurthi, Sondek, Hulihen, and Pedersen, 1992*c*; Chuang, Gittis, Abeygunawardana, Pedersen, and Mildvan, 1994) including circular dichroism spectroscopy and NMR, to relate structure to function. In addition, experiments are underway in an attempt to crystallize one of these nucleotide domains.

Work described here will focus specifically on the CFTR protein as mutations within both of its nucleotide domains have been linked to cystic fibrosis. Progress made in this laboratory in the study of these two nucleotide domains will be briefly described.

CFTR is an integral membrane protein (Riordan, Rommens, Kerem, Alon, Rozmahel, Grzelczak, Zilenski, Lok, Plausic, and Chow, 1989) comprised within a single polypeptide chain of 1,480 amino acids (Fig. 1). The five major domains include two nucleotide binding folds (NBF1 and NBF2), a regulatory domain (R), and two transmembrane spanning regions (TMSs). The latter, at least in part, form a Cl^- channel that is believed to require, for optimal function, both ATP hydrolysis

(Anderson, Berger, Rich, Gregory, Smith, and Welsh, 1991) mediated by NBF1 and phosphorylation of the R domain mediated by protein kinase A and/or other cellular kinases (Tabcharani, Chang, Riordan, Hanrahan, 1991; Cheng, Rich, Marshall, Gregory, Welsh, and Smith, 1991). Over 200 different mutations in the gene encoding CFTR induce amino acid changes in the protein which in turn cause cystic fibrosis (Tsui, 1992). Most cause mild forms of the disease, whereas others, like ΔF508 CFTR, result in severe forms of the disease. Unfortunately, ~90% of all cystic fibrosis patients have been reported to have at least one ΔF508 allele (Kerem, Corey, Kerem, Rommens, Mariewicz, Levinson, Tsui, and Durie, 1990).

NBF1 spans a ~155 amino acid region of CFTR (residues 433–588) and includes a Walker A (GX_4GKT/S), a Walker B ($RX_{6-8}h_4D$), and so-called linker or C consensus (LSXGXR/K). The Walker A and B consensus are found in many nucleotide binding proteins (Walker, Saraste, Runswick, and Gay, 1982) including adenylate kinases, ATP synthases, the RecA protein, and all members of the ABC transporter superfamily (Higgins, 1992). The C consensus, however, appears to be a unique feature of the ABC transporter superfamily (Shyamala, Baichwai, Beall, and Ames, 1991).

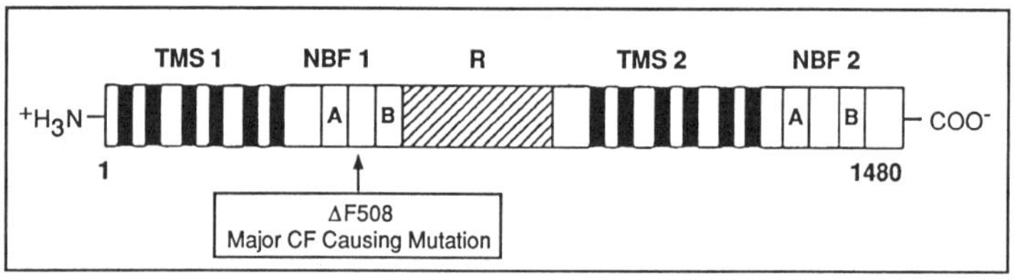

Figure 1. Presentation of the primary structure of the CFTR molecule. The relative positions of the five domains and the location of the ΔF508 mutation are depicted.

As no three-dimensional structural data is available for CFTR, or for any other member of the ABC transporter superfamily, NBF1 has been assumed to fold in a manner similar to adenylate kinase, the crystal structure of which is known (Schulz, Elzinga, Marx, and Schirmer, 1974; Sachsenheimer and Schulz, 1977). Fig. 2 *A* depicts the structural fold of adenylated kinase (Schulz et al., 1974; Sachsenheimer and Schulz, 1977). The region shown in black consisting of β strand/α helix/ β strand secondary structural organization is known to participate in binding ATP (Fry, Kuby, and Mildvan, 1986; Mildvan, 1986). Within this region the A consensus is located near the interface of the α helix and the loop (P loop). The A consensus is believed to interact directly with one or more of the three phosphate groups of ATP while the α helix may participate, in part, in binding the purine ribose moiety (Fry et al., 1986; Mildvan, 1989). The B consensus is located in a different region of adenylate kinase but, nevertheless, lies near the A consensus, and in some ATP binding proteins is believed to interact with Mg^{2+} (Story and Steitz, 1992).

Fig. 2 *A* shows also where the C consensus of NBF1 would be predicted to lie within the adenylate kinase fold. Significantly, its position resides downstream from the B consensus. Therefore, in three-dimensional space the A, B, and C consensus regions are predicted to lie near one another. The C consensus evidently does not contribute to nucleotide binding per se.

Of the 19 major mutations within NBF1 that cause cystic fibrosis (Tsui, 1992), it is interesting to note that 13 lie within or near consensus regions (Fig. 2 *B*). The remaining six mutations lie within or near a hydrophobic β-strand insert where the major disease causing mutation ΔF508 occurs. Although this region was originally believed to be α helical in character (Hyde, Gill, Hubbard, and Higgins, 1990), four different programs for predicting secondary structure have been shown more recently to report β-strand character (Thomas et al., 1991). It is possible that in the folding pathway, a β strand is first to form which is then converted to an α-helix in the

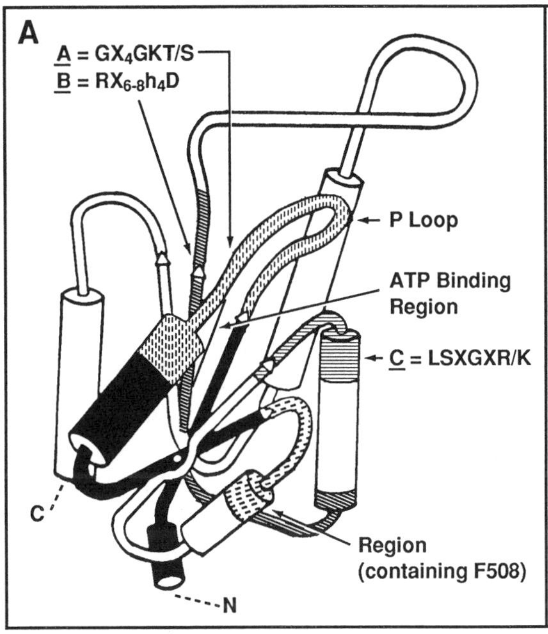

B

Mutation	Region
A455E	A
G458V	
L558S	B
A559T	
R560T	
Y563N	
P574H	
S549R	C
S549N	
S549I	
G551S	
G551D	
R553Q	
G480C	Near ΔF508
S492F	
E504Q	
ΔI507	
ΔF508	
V520F	

Figure 2. Adenylate kinaselike fold predicted in all members of the ABC transporter superfamily. Note the close proximity of the A, B, and C consensus to the ATP binding pocket, and CFTR to F508. Some investigators suggest that the rather hydrophobic insert containing F508 may interact with the membrane. (*B*) Mutations in NBF1 that cause cystic fibrosis. Boxes enclose mutations with consensus motifs.[1]

final folded structure. Whether or not this segment fits compactly within the adenylate kinaselike fold in NBF1 or projects out from it and into the membrane as speculated by some workers (Hyde et al., 1990; Baichwai, Liu, and Ames, 1993; Arispe, Rojas, Hartman, Sorscher, and Pollard, 1992) remains an interesting concept to be tested experimentally.

NBF2 spans a ~165 amino acid region of CFTR (residues 1219–1386) and includes the Walker A and Walker B consensus regions, as well as the C consensus.

[1] We are just completing the homology modeling of NBF1 and NBF2 in three dimensions based on known x-ray structures.

NBF2 exhibits considerable amino acid sequence homology to NBF1 (Smit, Wilkinson, Mansoura, Collins, and Dawson, 1993), and like NBF1, there are a number of mutations within the domain that result in cystic fibrosis (Tsui, 1992). However, none are as severe as that produced by the ΔF508 mutation in NBF1.

Results and Conclusions

In this section, experiments conducted over the past four years on the two nucleotide domains of the CFTR protein are briefly described. Experimental details and a more detailed discussion of most of this work can be found in (Ko et al., 1993, 1994; Thomas et al., 1991, 1992*b,c;* Thomas and Pedersen, 1993).

Preparations of NBF1 and NBF2 Peptides, and an NBF1 Fusion Protein

When we commenced this work, the CFTR protein had not been isolated, and there was no direct evidence that the two predicted nucleotide domains, NBF1 and NBF2

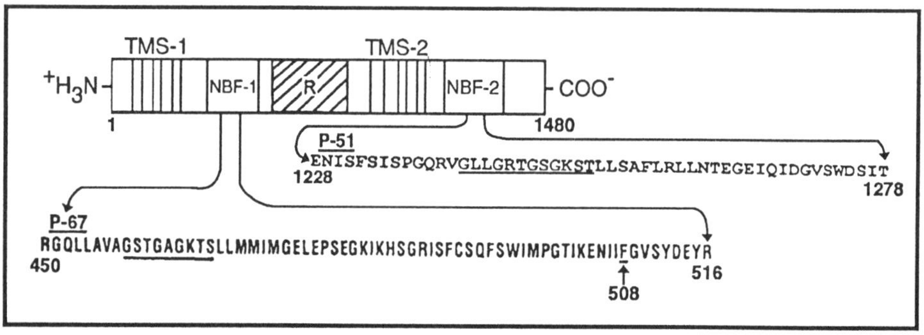

Figure 3. Peptides corresponding to the indicated regions of NBF1 and NBF2 of CFTR. These were chemically synthesized on a peptide synthesizer (model 430A, Applied Biosystems, Inc.) (Thomas et al., 1991; Ko et al., 1994). After hydrogen fluoride cleavage from the solid phase, the peptides were purified by reverse phase HPLC chromatography on a Waters C_{18} column. The Walker A consensus motif and F508 are underlined.

were in fact ATP binding domains. For this reason we designed, chemically synthesized, and purified both a 67 amino acid segment (P-67) of NBF1 (Thomas et al., 1991), which included the Walker A consensus motif and phenylalanine 508, and a 51 amino acid segment (P-51) of NBF2 (Ko et al., 1994) which also included the Walker A consensus motif (Fig. 3). These peptides correspond to the central core region of the adenylate kinase model where ATP is known to bind.

In addition to the above, we employed recombinant DNA technology to overexpress in *E. coli* the complete NBF1 domain (F433→S589) in fusion with the maltose binding protein (MBP) (Ko et al., 1993). The MBP protein was used both to facilitate purification on an amylose column and to provide a soluble MBP-NBF1 fusion product that might be suitable for crystallization. All three proteins, P-67, P-51 and MBP-NBF1, were subjected after preparation to a variety of purification tests as indicated in Table I. They were all judged to be >95% pure, and therefore, suitable for functional analysis.

Secondary structure. The three CFTR segments (P-67 from NBF1, MBP-NBF1, and P-51 from NBF2) were all shown by circular dichroism spectroscopy to exhibit significant secondary structure (Table II). Interestingly, the P-67 and P-51 peptides, which both span regions of NBF1 and NBF2 containing the Walker A consensus motif, distribute their secondary structural elements quite differently with P-67 exhibiting a high content of β-strand character relative to α helix and with P-51 exhibiting a high content of α-helical character relative to β strand. Neither P-67 nor P-51 showed an obvious propensity to form multimolecular structures, whereas the MBP-NBF1 construct, and not MBP alone, showed a propensity to form soluble organized polymeric structures which under high salt conditions partially dissociate and form microcrystals (see Fig. 8 of Ko et al., 1993). Clearly, a three-dimensional structure of the wild-type and ΔF508-NBF1 would be of particular significance in revealing the chemical details characterizing that region of NBF1 where the critical cystic fibrosis causing mutation lies. The formation of microcrystals of the MBP-NBF1 fusion protein represents an encouraging first step.

TABLE I
Yield and Criteria of Purity of NBF1 and NBF2 Components of CFTR

CFTR component	Region	Yield	Criteria of purity
P-67 from NBF1	R450 → P516	6–10 mg*	HPLC, SDS-PAGE, AA, and NH_2 terminus sequence analysis
MBP-MBF1	F433 → S589	~25 mg‡	HPLC, SDS-PAGE, AA, and NH_2 terminus sequence analysis
P-51 from NBF2	E1228 → T1278	6–10 mg*	HPLC, SDS-PAGE, AA, NH_2 terminus sequence and mass spectral analysis

*From ~300 mg of crude starting material.
‡Per liter cell culture.
AA, amino acid composition analysis.
See Ko et al. (1993, 1994) and Thomas et al. (1991) for details.

ATP binding. All of the above CFTR components prepared in this laboratory were found to bind the fluorescent nucleotide analogue trinitrophenyl-ATP (TNP-ATP) which could be displaced with ATP. Several control proteins including insulin failed to bind TNP-ATP. Table III shows that dissociation constants (K_ds) for ATP were all in the low mM range (0.30–1.8 mM) in analogy to numerous intracellular ATP-dependent enzymes. All CFTR components also bound TNP-ADP and to a much lesser extent TNP-AMP. Mg^{2+} was not necessary for nucleotide binding nor did it appreciably affect K_d values for all of the above CFTR components.

The studies described above demonstrate that NBF1 and NBF2 do interact with both ATP and ADP.

Effect of the ΔF508 mutation on the structure and function of the NBF1 peptide and on the MBP-NBF1 fusion protein. About 90% of all cystic fibrosis patients have been reported to have at least one ΔF508 CFTR allele (Chuang et al., 1994). Therefore, it was important to prepare and characterize the same NBF1 segments described above, i.e., P-67 and MBP-NBF1 but lacking phenylalanine 508. The following peptide called P-66 lacking F508 was prepared first employing a peptide synthesizer (model 430 A, Applied Biosystems, Inc., Foster City, CA) using again the same solid phase method used for P-67 (Thomas et al., 1991). No obvious problems were encountered in either the synthesis or subsequent reverse phase HPLC purification of P-66. A product judged >95% pure by SDS-PAGE, HPLC, amino acid, and sequence analysis was obtained. The yield was 6–10 mg from the crude starting material, in the same range as that obtained for the P-67 wild-type peptide. MBP-NBF1 lacking F508 was then prepared by PCR using the C-1-1/5 clone as the template (Ko et al., 1993). The fusion protein after overexpression in *E. coli*, was purified to apparent homogeneity on an amylose column. The yield of (ΔF508) MBP-NBF1 was ~25 mg/liter of cell culture, in the same range as that obtained for the MBP-NBF1 wild-type protein. The P-66 peptide lacking F508 and the (ΔF508) MBP-NBF1 construct were then analyzed in detail for structural and functional differences from the wild-type proteins.

P-66, physical characterization. The circular dichroism spectra presented in Fig. 4 *A* show clearly that the P-66 peptide bearing the ΔF508 mutation has less ordered structure than the wild-type P-67 peptide. Deconvolution of the two spectra using four different programs (Thomas et al., 1992*b*) indicated that deletion of F508

TABLE II
Relative Secondary Structural Elements of NBF1 and NBF2 Components of CFTR as Determined by Circular Dichroism Spectroscopy

CFTR component	Region	Secondary structural element*		
		α helix	β strand	Other‡
			% of total	
P-67 from NBF1	R450 → R516	<10	80	10–15
MBP-NBF1	F433 → S589	40	24	36
P-51 from NBF2	E1228 → T1278	20–28	6–11	61–74

*Deconvolution of the spectral data was carried out using the Prosec program.
‡Random coil + turns.
See Ko et al. (1993, 1994) and Thomas et al. (1991) for details.

from P-67 to give P-66 is accompanied by a loss of β-sheet secondary structure and a corresponding gain of random coil. Significantly, four different programs for predicting secondary structure indicate that F508 lies within a β-strand region (Thomas et al., 1991). Therefore, one of the simplest interpretations of these studies is that deletion of F508 destabilizes a β-sheet structure and unfolding occurs.

The circular dichroism experiments were reproduced in many different experiments and at many different dilutions of P-66 and P-67, and suggested that deletion of F508 produces a less stable peptide. For this reason we examined the effect of urea on the folding of P-67 and P-66, a study which revealed that the P-66 peptide bearing the F508 mutation unfolds (half maximally) at a significantly lower urea concentration (Fig. 4 *B*). In other studies not presented here, we have shown also that the P-66 peptide unfolds (half maximally) at a temperature 17° below that of P-67.

P-66, ATP binding. P-66 binds TNP-ATP as well as the wild-type peptide P-67. Thus, the localized disruption of structure within the F508 region evidently has little or no effect on the ATP binding region containing the Walker A consensus.

However, when nucleotide binding is measured in the presence of 4 M urea the wild-type peptide retains significant TNP-ATP binding capacity while the mutant peptide has lost this function (Thomas et al., 1992). It will be noted in Fig. 4 *B* that at 4 M urea the P-67 peptide retains about one third of its original secondary structure while the P-66 peptide is completely unfolded.

In other studies we found no detectable capacity for these peptides to catalyze the hydrolysis of ATP.

Model. The structural and functional studies on the wild-type P-67 and mutant P-66 peptides led us to consider the chemical and structural events that may take place when F508 is deleted from a β sheet region of CFTR. As illustrated in Fig. 5, one possibility is that a register shift will occur requiring reorientation of some amino acid side chains from one face of the β sheet to the other. Alternatively, a "β bulge" could form maintaining the residues on each face of the β sheet. Finally, neither of these new structures may be as stable as the original structure and, thus, will not spontaneously fold under physiological conditions. We believe that the latter possibility is most consistent with our structural and functional studies.

TABLE III
Relative Nucleotide-binding Properties of NBF1 and NBF2 Components of CFTR

CFTR component	Region	Dissociation constant (K_d) for ATP	Nucleotide specificity
		mM	
P-67 from NBF-1	R450 → R516	0.59	TNP-ATP > TNP-ADP > TNP-AMP
MBF-NBF1	F433 → S589	1.80	TNPATP > TNP-ADP > TNP-AMP
P-51 from NBF2	E1228 → T1278	0.46	TNP-ATP > TNP-ADP > TNP-AMP

See Ko et al. (1993, 1994) and Thomas et al. (1991) for details.

Hypothesis. Early studies on the membrane trafficking of intact CFTR within the cell were at first puzzling. Some investigators reported that the ΔF508 mutant protein underwent biosynthetic arrest and failed to travel to the plasma membrane (Rich, Anderson, Gregory, Cheng, Paul, Jefferson, McCann, Klinger, Smith, and Welsh, 1990; Anderson, Rich, Gregory, Smith, and Welsh, 1991; Denning, Ostegaard, and Welsh, 1992), whereas other workers reported that the mutant protein does travel to the plasma membrane in functional form (Li, Ramjeesingh, Reyers, Jensen, Chang, Rommens, and Bear, 1993; Drum, Wilkinson, Smit, Worrell, Strong, Frizzell, Dawson, and Collins, 1991). Our studies on purified components, which showed that the ΔF508 mutant peptide (P-66) is less stable, led us to propose that protein unfolding may be the molecular basis of most cases of cystic fibrosis (Thomas, Ko, and Pedersen, 1992*b*). Thus, we suggested that at 37° the ΔF508 mutant protein may be unstable and undergo biosynthetic arrest in some animal cells because of the inability to fold into a compact structure whereas at 27°, i.e., in insect cells (Sf9), the mutant protein may be able to refold into a stable functional protein and travel to the plasma membrane. (In the latter case, it is predicted that deletion of F508 would be accompanied by the formation of a "remodeled" β-sheet region, two possibilities of which are illustrated in Fig. 5).

Consistent with the above hypothesis Denning, Anderson, Amara, Marshall, Smith, and Welsh (1992) demonstrated that reduced temperature facilitates the processing of the ΔF508 CFTR in 3T3 fibroblasts and C127 cells, resulting in the appearance of cAMP-regulated Cl- channels in the plasma membrane. In a subsequent review (Thomas and Pedersen, 1993), we called attention to the possible use of chaperones in the treatment of cystic fibrosis.

(ΔF508) MBP-NBF1, physical and functional characterization. In a thorough study (Ko et al., 1993) we found no obvious differences in the physical and functional properties of wild-type MBP-NBF1 and (ΔF508) MBP-NBF1. These studies included (*a*) Secondary structural analysis by circular dichroism spectroscopy; (*b*) Susceptibility to protease digestion; (*c*) TNP-ATP binding and its competitive displacement by ATP; (*d*) Effect of urea on the nucleotide binding function; (*e*) HPLC molecular sieve chromatography; and (*f*) Propensity to form polymeric structures and microcrystals.

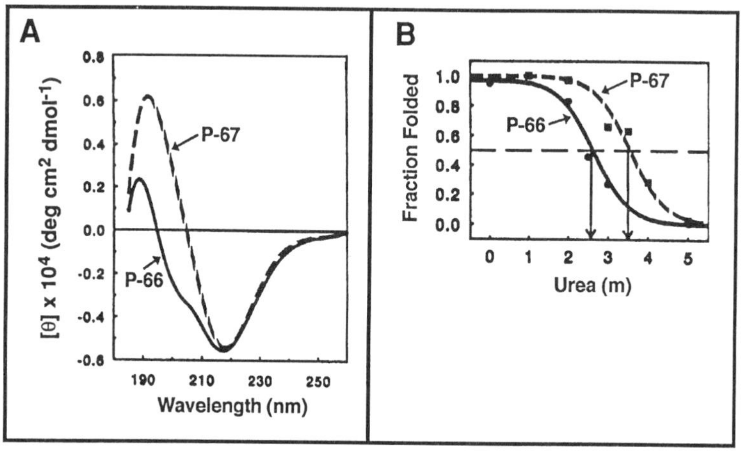

Figure 4. (*A*) Comparison of the circular dichroism spectra of the wild type and P-66 peptides indicating differences in secondary structure. The mean residue molar ellipticity is plotted vs wavelength (reprinted with permission, *Journal of Bioenergetics and Biomembranes*). (*B*) Comparison of the unfolding patterns of P-67 and P-66 in urea based on changes in the mean residue molar ellipticity at 218 nm and reflecting clear differences in the relative stabilities of the two peptides. (for details see Thomas et al., 1992*b*; Thomas and Pedersen, 1993).

These studies together with the additional finding that the maltose binding protein remains associated with NBF1 or ΔF508-NBF1 even after cleavage of the fusion junction, indicates that the obvious structural, stability, and functional differences between mutant and wild-type domains observed for the P-67 and P-66 peptides are not evident. This apparent discrepancy may be explained when one considers that P-67 and P-66 may represent folding intermediates on the pathway toward the native state while the MBP-NBF1 fusion proteins might be the finally folded structures in which the presence of one deleted amino acid fails to make a large difference. Therefore, if one were to obtain a crystal structure of the fusion proteins described here, it may be possible to deduce the minimal structural change that occurs when ΔF508 is deleted. We intend to work toward this goal.

Findings briefly summarized above are significant for several reasons. First, studies with P-67 and P-66 provided the first experimental evidence indicating that the major cystic fibrosis causing mutation, ΔF508, alters the structure and stability of NBF1. Secondly, these studies provide chemical insight into those changes that may take place in NBF1 when F508 is deleted. Thirdly, MBP or other proteins may be

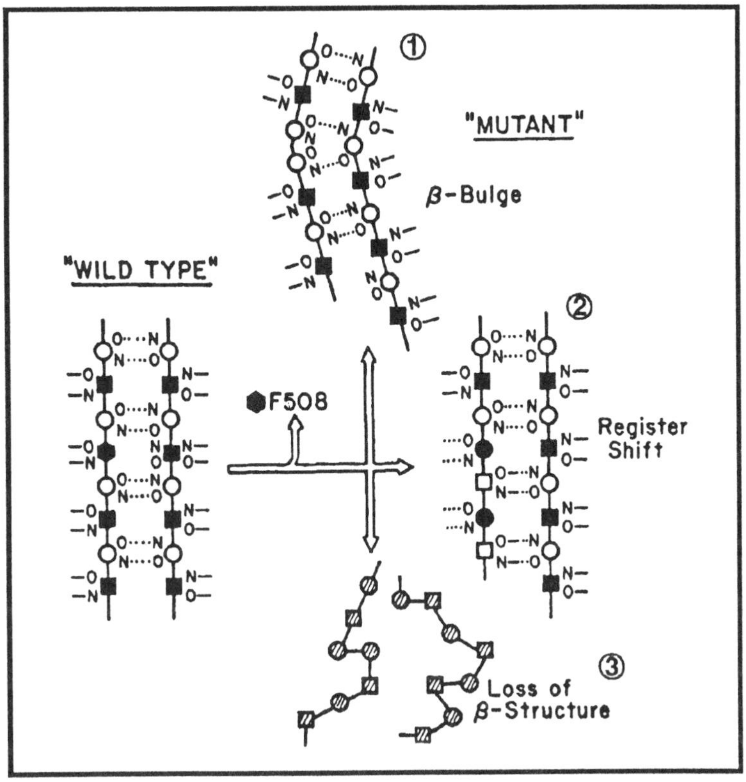

Figure 5. The possible effects of deleting F508 from a β-sheet region. (reprinted with permission from the *Journal of Biological Chemistry*). The β sheet may reform into either structure 1 or 2. However, if the latter are not thermodynamically stable structures, they would not form as depicted in 3. The experimental data obtained on the P-66 peptide relative to the control P-67 peptide indicate that possibility 3 is correct (Thomas et al., 1992*b*).

considered to minimize the effect of the deletion of F508 so that the mutant protein is more similar to that of the wild-type protein. Finally, studies with the MBP-NBF1 and (ΔF508) MBP-NBF1 fusion proteins have provided the first CFTR systems to date amenable to crystallization.

Other studies in progress. The folding pathway of CFTR is being studied in greater detail to define those components of the cell involved in this process. Also, studies are being conducted to establish whether NBF1 exhibits the capacity to hydrolyze ATP and to interact with biological membranes.

Acknowledgments

We are grateful to Dr. Wu-Schyong Liu for the synthesis of P-51. We are grateful also to Mrs. Jackie Seidl for processing the manuscript for publication.

Supported by National Institutes of Health grant DK 43962 to Peter L. Pedersen and by a grant from the Cystic Fibrosis Foundation. Young Hee Ko is the recipient of a New Investigator grant from the Cystic Fibrosis Foundation.

References

Anderson, M.P., H. A. Berger, D. P. Rich, R. J. Gregory, A. E. Smith, and M. J. Welsh. 1991. Nucleoside triphosphates are required to open the CFTR chloride channel. *Cell.* 67:775–784.

Anderson, M.P., D. P. Rich, R. J. Gregory, A. E. Smith, and M. J. Welsh. 1991. Generation of cAMP-activated chloride currents by expression of CFTR. *Science.* 251:679–682.

Arispe, N., E. Rojas, J. Hartman, E. J. Sorscher, and H. B. Pollard. 1992. Intrinsic anion channel activity of the recombinant first nucleotide binding fold of the cystic fibrosis transmembrane conductance regulator protein. *Proceedings of the National Academy of Sciences, USA.* 89:1539–1543.

Baichwal, V., D. Liu, and G. F.-L. Ames. 1993. The ATP-binding component of a prokaryotic traffic ATPase is exposed to the periplasmic (external) surface. *Proceedings of the National Academy of Sciences, USA.* 90:620–624.

Cheng, S. H., D. P. Rich, J. Marshall, R. J. Gregory, M. J. Welsh, and A. E. Smith. 1991. Phosphorylation of the R domain by cAMP-dependent protein kinase regulates the CFTR chloride channel. *Cell.* 66:1027–1036.

Chuang, W-J., A. G. Gittis, C. Abeygunawardana, P. L. Pedersen, and A. S. Mildvan. 1995. Solution structure of the metal-ATP-complex of PP-50 an ATP-binding peptide from F1-ATPase. *Archives of Biochemistry and Biophysics.* In press.

Denning, G., M. P. Anderson, J. F. Amara, J. Marshall, A. E. Smith, and M. J. Welsh. 1992. Processing of mutant cystic fibrosis transmembrane conductance regulator is temperature-sensitive. *Nature.* 358:761–764.

Denning, G.M., L. S. Ostedgaard, and M. J. Welsh. 1992. Abnormal localization of cystic fibrosis transmembrane conductance regulator in primary cultures of cystic fibrosis airway epithelia. *Journal of Cell Biology.* 118:551–559.

Doige, C. A., and G. Ferro-Luzzi Ames. 1993. ATP-dependent transport systems in bacteria and humans: relevance to cystic fibrosis and multidrug resistance. *Annual Review of Microbiology.* 47:291–319.

Drumm, M. L., D. J. Wilkinson, L. S. Smit, R. T. Worrell, T. V. Strong, R. A. Frizzell, D. C. Dawson, and F. S. Collins. 1991. Chloride conductance expressed by ΔF508 and other mutant CFTRs in *Xenopus* oocytes. *Science.* 254:1797–1800.

Fry, D. C., S. A. Kuby, and A. S. Mildvan. 1986. ATP-binding site of adenylate kinase: mechanistic implication of its homology with *Ras*-encoded p21, F1-ATPase, and other nucleotide binding properties. *Proceedings of the National Academy of Sciences, USA.* 83:907–911.

Garboczi, D.N., J. H. Hullihen, and P. L. Pedersen. 1988. Mitochondrial ATP synthase:

overexpression in *Escherichia coli* of a rat liver β-subunit peptide and its interaction with adenine nucleotides. *Journal of Biological Chemistry.* 263:15694–15698.

Garboczi, D.N., P. J. Thomas, and P. L. Pedersen. 1990. Rat liver mitochondrial ATP synthase. Effects of mutations in the glycine-rich region of a β-subunit peptide on its interaction with adenine nucleotides. *Journal of Biological Chemistry*. 265:14632–14637.

Higgins, C.F. 1992. ABC transporters: from microorganisms to man. *Annual Review of Cell Biology.* 8:67–113.

Hyde. S., P. Emsley, M. J. Hartshorn, M. M. Mimmack, U. Gileadi, S. R. Pearce, M. P. Gallagher, D. R. Gill, R. E. Hubbard, and C. F. Higgins. 1990. Structural model of ATP-binding proteins associated with cystic fibrosis, multidrug resistance, and bacterial transport. *Nature*. 346:362–365.

Kerem, E., M. Corey, B. S. Kerem, J. Rommens, D. Mariewicz, H. Levison, H., L.-C. Tsui, and P. Durie. 1990. The relationship between genotype and phenotype in cystic fibrosis analysis of the most common mutation (ΔF508). *New England Journal of Medicine.* 323:1517–1522.

Ko, Y.H., P. J. Thomas, and P. L. Pedersen. 1994. The cystic fibrosis transmembrane conductance regulator: nucleotide binding to a synthetic peptide segment from the second predicted nucleotide binding fold. *Journal of Biological Chemistry.* 269:14584–14588.

Ko, Y.H., P. J. Thomas, and P. L. Pedersen. 1993. The cystic fibrosis transmembrane conductance regulator: overexpression, purification, and characterization of wild-type and F508 mutant forms of the first nucleotide binding fold in fusion with the maltose-binding protein. *Journal of Biological Chemistry.* 268:24330–24338.

Lee, J. H., D. N. Garboczi, P. J. Thomas, and P.L. Pedersen. 1990. Mitochondrial ATP synthase: cDNA cloning, amino acid sequence, overexpression, and properties of the rat liver β subunit. *Journal of Biological Chemistry.* 265:4664–4669.

Li. C., M. Ramjeesingh, E. Reyers, T. Jensen, X. Chang, J. M. Rommens, and C. E. Bear. 1993. The cystic fibrosis mutation (ΔF508) does not influence the chloride channel activity of CFTR. *Nature Genetics.* 3:311–316.

Mildvan, A. S. 1989. Studies of the interaction of substrates with enzymes and their peptide fragments. *FASEB Journal*. 3:1705–1714.

Pedersen, P. L., and L. M. Amzel. 1993. ATP synthases: structure, reaction center, mechanisms, and regulation of one of nature's most unique machines. *Journal of Biological Chemistry.* 268:9937–9940.

Rich, D. P., M. P. Anderson, R. J. Gregory, S. H. Cheng, S. Paul, D. M. Jefferson, J. D. McCann, K. W. Klinger, A. E. Smith, and M. J. Welsh. 1990. Expression of cystic fibrosis transmembrane conductance regulator corrects defective chloride channel regulation in cystic fibrosis airway epithelial cells. *Nature.* 347:358–363.

Riordan, J. R., J. M. Rommens, B. Kerem, N. Alon, R. Rozmahel, Z. Grzelczak, J. Zielenski, S. Lok, N. Plausic, and J. L. Chow. 1989. Identification of the cystic fibrosis gene: cloning and characterization of complementary DNA. *Science*. 245:1066–1073.

Sachsenheimer, W., and G. E. Schulz. 1977. Two conformations of crystalline adenylate kinase. *Journal of Biological Cemistry.* 114:23–36.

Schulz, G.E., M. Elzinga, F. Marx, and R. H. Schirmer. 1974. Three-dimensional structure of adenylate kinase. *Nature.* 250:120–123.

Shyamala, V., V. Baichwal, E. Beall, and G. F. Ames. 1991. Structure function analysis of the histidine permease and comparison with cystic fibrosis mutations. *Journal of Biological Chemistry.* 266:18714–18719.

Smit, L.S., D. J. Wilkinson, M. K. Mansoura, F. S. Collins, and D. C. Dawson. 1993. Functional roles of the nucleotide-binding folds in the activation of the cystic fibrosis transmembrane conductance regulator. *Proceedings of the National Academy of Sciences, USA.* 90:9963–9967.

Story, R.M., and T. A. Steitz. 1992. Structure of the RecA protein-ADP complex. *Nature.* 355:374–376.

Tabcharani, J. A., X. -B. Chang, J. R. Riordan, and J. W. Hanrahan. 1991. Phosphorylation-regulated Cl^- channel in CHO cells stably expressing the cystic fibrosis gene. *Nature.* 352:628–631.

Thomas, P.J., and P. L. Pedersen. 1993. Effects of the ΔF508 mutation on the structure, function, and folding of the first nucleotide-binding domain of CFTR. *Journal of Bioenergetics and Biomembranes.* 25:11–19.

Thomas, P. J., D. N. Garboczi, and P. L. Pedersen. 1992*a*. Mutational analysis of the consensus nucleotide binding sequences in the rat liver mitochondrial ATP synthase β-subunit. *Journal of Biological Chemistry.* 267: 20331–20338.

Thomas, P.J., Y. H. Ko., and P. L. Pedersen. 1992*b*. Altered protein folding may be the molecular basis of most cases of cystic fibrosis. *FEBS Letters.* 312:7–9.

Thomas, P.J., P. Shenbagamurthi, J. Sondek, J. M. Hullihen, and P. L. Pedersen. 1992. The cystic fibrosis transmembrane conductance regulator: effects of the most common cystic fibrosis-causing mutations on the secondary structure and stability of a synthetic peptide. *Journal of Biological Chemistry.* 267:5727–5730.

Thomas, P.J., P. Shenbagamurthi, X. Ysern, and P. L. Pedersen. 1991. Cystic fibrosis transmembrane conductance regulator: nucleotide binding to a synthetic peptide. *Science.* 251:555–557.

Tsui, L.-C. 1992. The spectrum of cystic fibrosis mutations. *Trends in Genetics.* 8:392–398.

Walker, J.E., M. Saraste, M. J. Runswick, and N. J. Gay. 1982. Distantly related sequences in the α- and β-subunits of ATP synthase, myosin, kinases, and other ATP-requiring enzymes and a common nucleotide binding fold. *EMBO Journal.* 1:945–951.

Chapter 2

Potassium Channel Disorders: Lessons from the *Shaker* Gene

New Potassium Channel Gene Families in Flies and Mammals: From Mutants to Molecules

Barry Ganetzky,* Jeffrey W. Warmke,‡ Gail Robertson,§ and Leo Pallanck*

**Laboratory of Genetics, and §Department of Physiology, University of Wisconsin, Madison, Wisconsin 53706; and ‡Department of Genetics and Molecular Biology, Merck Research Laboratories, Rahway, New Jersey 07065*

Introduction

Of the various strategies that have been utilized for molecular analysis of ion channel polypeptides and the genes that encode them, the genetic approach has proven to be one of the most powerful (Ganetzky and Wu, 1986; Wu and Ganetzky, 1992). Among metazoans, this approach has been limited almost exclusively to *Drosophila* because of the sophisticated genetic, cytogenetic, and molecular tools available for use with this organism. These techniques make it relatively easy to screen large numbers of mutagenized flies for all the genes capable of mutating to confer a particular phenotype. Furthermore, once a mutant gene has been identified, its precise location on the giant polytene chromosomes can be readily determined. Several different strategies can then be used to clone the gene of interest starting only with the knowledge of its cytological location (Rubin, 1988). In addition to its excellence for genetic studies, *Drosophila* is well suited for many types of electrophysiological analyses as well. This has made it possible to combine genetic, electrophysiological, and molecular techniques to study ion channels in this organism.

The premise of this approach is that the genes encoding ion channels can be identified and subsequently cloned via mutations in these genes. In practice, this involves isolating various types of behavioral mutants and screening for those with conspicuous electrophysiological defects, particularly in the neuromuscular system of larvae and adults, which is most accessible for experimental analysis (Jan and Jan, 1976; Wu, Ganetzky, Jan, Jan, and Benzer, 1978; Tanouye and Wyman, 1980). The advantage of this genetic strategy is that it provides an unbiased way of identifying genes that encode ion channels or that otherwise affect channel function or regulation in the absence of any prior biochemical information about the encoded polypeptide and irrespective of its relative abundance or scarcity. Mutations can thus provide experimental handles for molecular isolation of genes encoding known proteins that are otherwise inaccessible; more important, they can lead to the discovery of new proteins. Although the genetic approach to ion channel genes has been limited to *Drosophila,* the results have not: ion channel polypeptides tend to be well conserved evolutionarily, so isolation of the relevant genes in *Drosophila* offers a direct route for isolation of the corresponding genes from most other organisms including humans.

The analysis of the *Shaker* (*Sh*) locus (Kaplan and Trout, 1969; Jan, Jan, and Dennis, 1977) provides a good illustration of these points. Until recently, biochemical purification of potassium channel polypeptides had not been achieved precluding molecular analysis via this route. However, molecular characterization of the *Sh* locus, mutations of which were known to eliminate a particular voltage-activated potassium current, revealed that it was likely to encode a component of potassium channels (Kamb, Iverson, and Tanouye, 1987; Tempel, Papazian, Schwarz, Jan, and Jan, 1987; Pongs, Kecskemethy, Muller, Krah-Jentgens, Baumann, Kiltz, Canal, Llamazares, and Ferrus, 1988). This conclusion was confirmed by functional expression of *Sh* cDNAs in *Xenopus* oocytes (Iverson, Tanouye, Lester, Davidson, and Rudy, 1988; Timpe, Jan, and Jan, 1988). Thus, *Sh* was the first potassium channel gene cloned from any organism. Subsequently three additional genes representing different subfamilies of potassium channels related to *Sh* were cloned from *Drosophila* on the basis of their homology with *Sh* probes (Salkoff, Baker, Butler, Covarrubias, Pak, and Wei, 1992). Homologues of each of these potassium channel genes have now been cloned from many different species including mammals (Strong, Chandy, and Gutman, 1993).

Although these studies of *Sh* and its relatives initiated the molecular analysis of potassium channels, the homology screens used to clone additional potassium channel genes was biased in favor of those sharing substantial similarity with the *Sh* family. Other types of potassium channel genes, which might be only distantly related to *Sh,* were unlikely to be recovered in such screens. For example, genes encoding calcium-activated potassium channels were not among those recovered as *Sh* homologues. Nonetheless, genes encoding other types of potassium channels could still be uncovered via appropriate mutations in *Drosophila* independent of any assumptions about sequence relationships. Because we had already identified mutations of two other genes, slowpoke (*slo*) and ether à go-go (*eag*), which had defects in potassium currents not affected by *Sh,* we pursued the molecular isolation of these genes. We review here the results of those studies leading to identification of two previously uncharacterized types of potassium channel polypeptides in flies and mammals.

A Mutation that Eliminates a Calcium-activated Potassium Current

The recessive, third chromosome mutation, *slo,* was discovered on the basis of its sluggish and uncoordinated phenotype (Elkins, Ganetzky, and Wu, 1986). Electrophysiological studies showed that repolarization of action potentials in flight muscles of *slo* homozygotes is ~10 times slower than normal (Elkins et al. 1986; Elkins and Ganetzky, 1988). Subsequently, voltage clamp experiments demonstrated that the basic defect is the complete and specific elimination of a fast, calcium-activated potassium current (I_{CF}) in muscles of both adults and larvae (Elkins et al., 1986; Komatsu, Singh, Rathe, and Wu, 1990). Alteration in evoked synaptic currents in *slo* mutants suggests that an I_{CF}-type current is also present in presynaptic motor terminals of *Drosophila* and is required for their normal repolarization (Gho and Ganetzky, 1992). The electrophysiological studies of *slo* mutants demonstrate that normal activity of *slo* is essential for the production or function of the I_{CF} type of calcium-activated potassium channels. However, these results did not establish whether *slo* actually encoded a component of these channels or perturbed their activity by some other mechanism. To resolve this question, we undertook molecular analysis of the *slo* locus (Atkinson, Robertson, and Ganetzky, 1991).

Molecular Analysis of *slo* Indicates It Encodes a Structural Component of Calcium-activated Potassium Channels

The gene was mapped cytologically to polytene band 96A17 on the salivary chromosomes by analysis of newly generated *slo* alleles associated with chromosome rearrangements. Genomic DNA from the region defined by the breakpoints of the rearrangements was cloned by chromosome jumping and walking. Localization of the breakpoints on the molecular map of the cloned region by Southern blot analysis and chromosomal in situ hybridization defined an approximate position of the *slo* transcription unit. A set of overlapping cDNAs corresponding to the *slo* transcript was identified by screening a head cDNA library with genomic probes from this region.

Sequence analysis revealed that the *slo* transcript encodes a polypeptide ~ 1,200 amino acids in length with seven hydrophobic domains near the amino terminus, reminiscent of the structure of potassium channel polypeptides in the *Sh* family. Each of the hydrophobic segments in the *slo* sequence has significant amino acid similarity with the corresponding segment of a *Sh*-family consensus sequence. The sixth hydrophobic segment, corresponding to the pore domain (Durell and Guy, 1992), is especially well conserved: in this region there are 11 identities and 5 conservative substitutions relative to the *Sh*-family consensus sequence in a region of 25 amino acids. 9 of the identities fall within a 12 amino acid segment that also contains 3 conservative substitutions. The fourth hydrophobic segment, corresponding to the S4 domain involved in voltage-dependent activation of members of the *Sh* family (Durell and Guy, 1992), is also strongly conserved. For all of the hydrophobic segments taken together there are 25% amino acid identities and 20% conservative substitutions in the alignment of the *slo* and *Sh* polypeptides. The similarity between the *slo* polypeptide and members of the *Sh* family of voltage-activated potassium channels indicates that they are derived from a common ancestor. However, there is sufficient divergence between the hydrophobic core regions of the *slo* polypeptide and all members of the extended *Sh* family of potassium channel subunits to indicate that *slo* is not another member of the *Sh* family but defines a distinct type of potassium channel polypeptide. Thus, on the basis of functional evidence indicating that *slo* mutations eliminate a calcium-activated potassium current in vivo together with structural evidence demonstrating the relationship of *slo* with known potassium channel subunits, it was apparent that *slo* encodes a component of calcium-activated potassium channels (Atkinson et al., 1991). Functional expression of calcium-activated potassium channels in *Xenopus* oocytes after injection of mRNA transcribed in vitro from *slo* cDNAs indicates that *slo* polypeptides can assemble in homomultimeric fashion to form these channels (Adelman, Shen, Kavanaugh, Warren, Wu, Lagrutta, Bond, and North, 1992).

Isolation of Mammalian Homologues of *slo*

Because of their large single-channel conductance (Komatsu et al., 1990; Adelman et al., 1992) *slo*-encoded channels appear to be the *Drosophila* equivalent of mammalian high conductance or BK-type of calcium-activated potassium channels. Strong, evolutionary conservation of the amino acid sequence of other ion channel polypeptides between flies and mammals suggested that probes from the *Drosophila slo* locus could be used to isolate mammalian counterparts. As expected, screens of mammalian cDNA libraries with *slo* cDNA probes resulted in the isolation of mouse (Butler, Tsunoba, McCobb, Wei, and Salkoff, 1993; Pallanck and Ganetzky, 1994) and human (Pallanck and Ganetzky, 1994) homologues of *slo* expressed in brain and skeletal muscle. So far, only a single *slo* homologue has been identified in mouse (*mslo*) and human (*hslo*) suggesting that other genes encoding calcium-activated potassium channels in these organisms, which are likely to be present, are probably structurally distinct from *slo.* In addition, considerable diversity of calcium-activated potassium channels appears to be generated in vivo by extensive alternative splicing of *slo* transcripts in *Drosophila* (Atkinson et al., 1991; Adelman et al., 1992), mouse (Butler et al., 1993) and human (Pallanck and Ganetzky, 1994) tissues.

Because mammalian BK channels are involved in a number of physiological activities (Rudy, 1988), mutations in a gene encoding a structural component of these channels would be expected to have profound phenotypic consequences. As a background for determining whether any human genetic diseases are associated with mutations in *hslo,* we mapped the chromosome location of this gene. This was facilitated by use of a panel of human-hamster hybrid cell lines each of which contained one of the 24 different human chromosomes. Oligonucleotide primers that specifically amplified a short fragment of the human *hslo* genomic sequence were used to assay each of the cell lines. The amplification product was detected only in the cell line containing chromosome 10 indicating that *hslo* maps to this chromosome (Pallanck and Ganetzky, 1994).

Calcium Sensitivity of Calcium-activated Potassium Channels Expressed from *mslo* cDNAs in *Xenopus* Oocytes Is Enhanced by an Additional Subunit

Although injection of either *slo* or *mslo* RNAs into *Xenopus* oocytes leads to expression of calcium-activated potassium channels (Adelman et al., 1992; Butler et al., 1993), the calcium concentration required to activate these channels is substantially higher than that required to activate the corresponding channels in vivo, suggesting that other factors are influencing the activity of these channels in their native environment. Recent biochemical purification of calcium-activated potassium channels from bovine tracheal smooth muscle demonstrates that these channels are composed of two subunits: an α-subunit homologous to the *Drosophila slo* polypeptide and a newly identified β-subunit distinct from other known potassium channel polypeptides (Knaus, Folander, Garcia-Calvo, Garcia, Kaczorowski, Smith, and Swanson, 1994). Although expression of the β-subunit alone in *Xenopus* oocytes does not produce functional channels, coexpression of the β-subunit with an α-subunit (*mslo*) results in the formation of heteromeric channels that are more sensitive to activation by voltage and calcium than channels composed of the α-subunit alone (McManus, Helms, Pallanck, Ganetzky, Swanson, and Leonard, 1994). The calcium concentration required to produce a channel open probability of 0.5 at 0 mV is reduced from 30 to 3 μM by coexpression of the β-subunit together with the α-subunit. Thus, coexpression of α- and β-subunits in *Xenopus* oocytes results in the formation of calcium-activated potassium channels whose calcium sensitivity resembles that of native BK channels in brain and smooth muscle. These results indicate that BK channels most likely function as heteromeric assemblies in vivo, at least in some cell types. Differential expression of the β-subunit could provide one mechanism for modifying the properties of BK channels in vivo.

The *eag* Mutation Defines Another Candidate Gene for Potassium Channels in *Drosophila*

Another potassium channel gene first characterized in *Drosophila* is the *eag* locus. Like *Sh, eag* was discovered because of its ether-sensitive leg-shaking phenotype (Kaplan and Trout, 1969). However, *eag* was not studied intensively until more than ten years later when it was rediscovered as a second-site mutation that interacted in striking synergistic fashion in double mutant combinations with *Sh* mutations (Ganetzky and Wu, 1983). In the larval neuromuscular preparation, *eag* mutations cause a high frequency of spontaneous action potentials that evoke synaptic potentials whose amplitude and duration are significantly increased relative to wild type (Ganetzky and Wu, 1983, 1985). In *eag Sh* double mutants, large, plateauing synaptic potentials are generated that last for up to 500 ms and are associated with equally long bursts of spikes in motor axons (Ganetzky and Wu, 1983, 1985). These phenotypes are qualitatively more extreme than the most severe defects observed in *eag* or *Sh* alone. The neuronal hyperexcitability associated with loss-of-function *eag* mutations suggested a possible defect in potassium currents. This interpretation could also account for the synergistic interaction between *eag* and *Sh* if the potassium current(s) affected by *eag* differed from the one affected by *Sh.* If that were true, the phenotype of the double mutant could be ascribed to simultaneous reduction or elimination of two or more different potassium currents with overlapping functions in the repolarization of nerve terminals. In voltage clamp studies, the amplitudes of four different potassium currents are apparently reduced in larval muscles of different *eag* alleles, providing direct evidence for an effect of this gene on potassium channels (Wu, Ganetzky, Liu, and Haugland, 1983; Zhong and Wu, 1991).

Molecular Analysis of *eag* Indicates It Encodes a Novel Potassium Channel Polypeptide

Molecular characterization of *eag* was undertaken to elucidate its effect on potassium currents. Procedures analogous to those described above for *slo* were used to clone *eag* genomic and cDNAs (Drysdale, Warmke, Kreber, and Ganetzky, 1991). *eag* was localized cytologically to polytene bands 13A2-5 on the salivary chromosome map and genomic DNA from this region was cloned. cDNAs corresponding to the *eag* transcript were isolated by screening head libraries with genomic probes from the region defined by *eag* breakpoint mutations. The polypeptide encoded by these cDNAs is 1,174 amino acids in length containing seven hydrophobic domains in the amino-terminal half of the sequence (Warmke, Drysdale, and Ganetzky, 1991). Each of these domains shares significant similarity in alignments with corresponding segments of a *Sh*-family consensus sequence. The regions of strongest conservation are in the fourth and sixth hydrophobic segments corresponding to the S4 and pore domains, respectively, of known potassium channel polypeptides (Durell and Guy, 1992). Overall, the membrane-spanning segments and the pore region of *eag* share 25% amino acid identities and 20% conserved substitutions with a *Sh*-family consensus sequence. The sequence similarity of the *eag* polypeptide in key functional regions with other known potassium channel polypeptides, together with the in vivo effects of *eag* mutations on membrane excitability and potassium currents, suggested that *eag* also encodes a structural component of potassium channels.

Although sequence comparisons clearly indicate a relationship between *eag* and members of the *Sh*-family of potassium channel genes, its divergence from all known members of this family exceeds that of the most distantly related members of this family indicating that *eag* encodes a distinct type of ion channel polypeptide. This conclusion is given further weight by additional sequence comparisons revealing that the *eag* polypeptide is, in fact, more closely related to polypeptides of cyclic nucleotide-gated cation (cNGC) channels present in vertebrate photoreceptors and olfactory epithelial (Kaupp, 1991) than to those of voltage-gated potassium channels in the *Sh* family (Guy, Durell, Warmke, Drysdale, and Ganetzky, 1991). However, the closest relatives of *eag* are the recently characterized *KAT1* and *AKT1* inwardly rectifying potassium channels of *Arabidopsis* (Anderson, Huprikar, Kochian, Lucas, and Gaber, 1992; Schachtman, Schroeder, Lucas, Anderson, and Gaber, 1992; Sentenac, Bonneaud, Minet, Lacroute, Salmon, Gaymard, and Grignon, 1992; Warmke and Ganetzky, 1994). The similarity between *eag*, cNGC channels, and the plant inwardly rectifying channels includes numerous identities distributed throughout the hydrophobic core and extends beyond the last hydrophobic segment into the carboxy-terminal region encompassing a segment homologous to the cyclic nucleotide binding domain (cNBD) of cyclic nucleotide binding proteins (Warmke and Ganetzky, 1994).

eag cCNAs Expressed in *Xenopus* Oocytes Mediate Voltage-activated, Potassium-selective, Outward Currents

The sequence similarity of *eag* with cNGC channels, whose gating is voltage independent but requires cyclic nucleotide binding and which are nonselective among monovalent cations, as well as with the *AKT1* and *KAT1* channels, which mediate an inward potassium current in response to membrane hyperpolarization, raises questions about the functional properties of *eag* channels. These questions are especially pertinent because the *eag* polypeptide has not yet been definitively associated with a particular channel type in vivo. Expression studies in *Xenopus* oocytes demonstrate that the *eag* polypeptide can assemble in homomeric fashion to form channels that pass an outward current in response to membrane depolarization (Robertson, Warmke, and Ganetzky, 1993; Bruggeman, Pardo, Stuhmer, and Pongs, 1993, Robertson, Warmke, and Ganetzky, unpublished results). Outward currents activate at ~ -40 mV and increase in amplitude at more positive potentials. The *eag* current contains two kinetically distinct components—a large early inactivating component and a smaller steady state component (Robertson et al., 1993). Hyperpolarizing command pulses from the holding potential of -80 mV do not evoke currents. Instantaneous *I–V* relationships determined from the analysis of tail currents evoked at a constant potential from various prepulse voltages show that gating of *eag* channels is voltage dependent. The *eag* channels are highly selective for potassium over sodium ions as judged by measurement of reversal potentials in different external potassium concentrations. In excised macropatches, the gating and kinetic characteristics of *eag* currents are maintained in the absence of cAMP or cGMP in the bath (Robertson et al., 1993). Although a small increase in current amplitude in the presence of cAMP has been reported (Bruggerman et al., 1993), the gating of *eag* channels clearly do not require cyclic nucleotides. These results demonstrate that *eag* channels are functionally quite distinct from either of their closest relatives, the inwardly rectifying channels of plants or the vertebrate cNGC channels. Instead, the gating and permeation properties of *eag* channels more closely resemble those of *Sh*-type potassium channels despite their more distant phylogenetic relationship to this family.

eag Is the Founding Member of a New Family of Potassium Channel Genes in Flies and Mammals

Voltage-activated ion channels are typically members of evolutionarily conserved multigene families (Strong et al., 1993). The discovery that *eag* encodes a voltage-activated potassium channel distinct from those encoded by *Sh* and its relatives suggested the possibility that *eag* is itself the prototype of a new potassium channel gene family analogous to the *Sh* family. To explore this possibility, we used low stringency hybridization and degenerate PCR screens to search for relatives of *eag* expressed in *Drosophila* and mammalian tissues (Warmke and Ganetzky, 1994; Warmke, Titus, and Ganetzky, unpublished results). Four additional genes have now been identified—one each in *Drosophila* (*elk*), mouse (*m-eag*), rat (*r-elk*), and human (*h-erg*). The polypeptides encoded by these genes clearly constitute a closely related family. Family members all share ~47% amino acid identity in their hydrophobic cores and all contain a segment homologous to the cNBD. Higher levels of identity between particular polypeptide pairs suggests the existence of at least three subfamilies. For example, the alignment of the *eag* and *m-eag* polypeptides in the region from the initiating methionine through the cNBD region contains 68% amino acid identities compared with ~45% identities for pairwise comparisons with other family members. Thus, *eag* and *m-eag* appear to represent counterpart genes in *Drosophila* and mouse respectively and define one subfamily. Similarly, the *elk* and *r-elk* polypeptides, which share 60% amino acid identities through the cNBD region, define a second subfamily. The *h-erg* polypeptide is equidistant from the *eag* and *elk* subfamilies (~43–47% identities) and thus appears not to be the human counterpart of either eag or elk but to define a third subtype of the *eag* family. We anticipate the identification of other genes corresponding to the human counterparts of *eag* and *elk* as well as a *Drosophila* counterpart of *h-erg*.

Consistent with the structural similarity of *m-eag* and *eag* polypeptides, expression of *m-eag* in *Xenopus* oocytes produces currents with properties similar to those mediated by *eag* channels (Robertson et al., 1994). The major difference is that the *m-eag* currents do not exhibit the inactivating component seen with *eag*. It will be of interest to express the channels encoded by *elk* and *h-erg* to see how their properties compare with those of the *eag* subfamily.

Strong conservation of the *eag* family from *Drosophila* to mammals suggests that in vivo functions are likely to be preserved as well. The striking hyperexcitability in *Drosophila* neurons caused by loss of *eag* function demonstrates the importance of *eag* channels in membrane repolarization. If *h-erg* has a similarly important function in the human nervous system, mutations of it would be predicted to lead to a marked neurological disorder such as those associated with seizures. To initiate linkage studies we mapped the chromosome location of *h-erg* by using a PCR-based assay to assay its presence or absence in a panel of human-hamster hybrid cell lines each carrying a known subset of human chromosomes (Warmke and Ganetzky, 1994).

Only human chromosome 7 showed perfect concordance for the *h-erg* PCR product, demonstrating that *h-erg* is located on this chromosome.

Discussion

These studies along with the previous characterization of *Sh* demonstrate the enormous power of using mutations affecting membrane excitability in *Drosophila* as a means of identifying genes encoding components of ion channels. This strategy paved the way for the first molecular analysis of three different families of potassium channel polypeptides represented by the *Sh, slo,* and *eag* genes and enabled isolation of closely related genes from other organisms, including humans.

In the case of *Sh* and *slo,* although the potassium channel types specified by these genes had been previously defined by electrophysiological and biophysical techniques, mutations provided the essential starting material for molecular studies. With *eag* the situation is different and in some respects even more surprising. Before the cloning and molecular analysis of *eag,* the channels defined by this gene were unknown. In fact, channels containing polypeptides encoded by *eag* family members still await electrophysiological description in vivo. Thus, *eag* represents the first instance where genetic analysis led to the discovery of an entirely new class of ion channels.

The discovery of the *eag* family of voltage-gated potassium channels reveals that potassium channel diversity in vivo is even greater than what has been inferred from the analysis of the extended *Sh* family. It will be of interest to determine the physiological roles of the *eag* family of potassium channels in vivo. The phenotype of *eag* mutations in *Drosophila* indicates that at least some members of this family are important for limiting neuronal excitability. Examination of the amino acid sequences and functional properties of channels encoded by the *eag* family with their closest known relatives, the plant inward rectifiers and the vertebrate cNGC channels, and their more distant relatives, the *Sh* family of voltage-activated potassium channels, will provide new opportunities to elucidate structure-function relationships in this ion channel superfamily. The *eag* family may also hold clues to the evolutionary relationships within this superfamily. The similarity of *eag* to the plant inward rectifiers, including an especially well-conserved segment in the pore region and a segment homologous to cNBDs, demonstrates that these features are ancient, predating the evolutionary divergence of plants and animals. Perhaps *eag*-type channels represent an ancestral form of voltage-activated potassium channels.

As demonstrated in the studies reviewed here, work in *Drosophila* has been of fundamental importance in identifying genes encoding ion channel polypeptides and in elucidating the primary structure of these molecules. Despite the progress in this area, many questions concerning the mechanisms that regulate the expression, assembly, subcellular localization, and modulation of ion channels in vivo await resolution. The same combination of genetics, electrophysiology, and molecular biology in *Drosophila* that has proven so powerful in identifying novel ion channel genes should prove equally useful in elucidating these aspects of channel regulation. Because perturbations in nervous system function, including those manifested as disease phenotypes in humans, are likely to result from genetic defects affecting the regulation of ion channels in addition to those affecting their structure, this knowledge will be of medical as well as scientific importance.

Acknowledgements

We thank Robert Kreber and Steven Titus for technical assistance.

Work reviewed here has been supported by a Klingenstein Fellowship, a McKnight Neurosciences Development Award, and grants from the NIH, the Markey Charitable Trust, the American Heart Association of Wisconsin, the Muscular Dystrophy Association, and the American Cancer Society.

References

Adelman, J., K.-Z. Shen, M. P. Kavanaugh, R. A., Warren, Y.-N. Wu, A. Lagrutta, C. T. Bond, and R. A. North. 1992. Calcium-activated potassium channels expressed from cloned complementary DNAs. *Neuron.* 9:209–216.

Anderson, J. A., S. S. Huprikar, L. V. Kochian, W. J. Lucas, and R. F. Gaber. 1992. Functional expression of a probable *Arabadopsis thaliana* potassium channel in *Saccharomyces cerevisiae. Proceedings of the National Academy of Sciences, USA.* 89:3736–3740.

Atkinson, N., G. Robertson, and B. Ganetzky. 1991. A structural component of calcium-activated potassium channels encoded by the *Drosophila slo* locus. *Science.* 253:551–555.

Bruggeman, A., L. A. Pardo, W. Stuhmer, and O. Pongs. 1993. Ether à go-go encodes a voltage-gated channel permeable to K^+ and Ca^{2+} and modulated by cAMP. *Nature.* 365:445–448.

Butler, A., S. Tsunoda, D. P. McCobb, A. Wei, and L. Salkoff. 1993. *mSlo,* a complex mouse gene encoding "maxi" calcium-activated potassium channels. *Science.* 261:221–224.

Drysdale, R. A., J. W. Warmke, R. Kreber, and B. Ganetzky. 1991. Molecular characterization of *eag,* a gene affecting potassium channels in *Drosophila. Genetics.* 127:497–505.

Durell, S. R., and H. R. Guy. 1992. Atomic scale structure and functional models of voltage-gated potassium channels. *Biophysical Journal.* 62:238–250.

Elkins, T., and B. Ganetzky. 1988. The roles of potassium currents in *Drosophila* flight muscles. *Journal of Neuroscience.* 8:428–434.

Elkins, T., B. Ganetzky, and C.-F. Wu. 1986. A *Drosophila* mutation that eliminates a calcium-dependent potassium current. *Proceedings of the National Academy of Sciences, USA.* 83:8415–8419.

Ganetzky, B., and C.-F. Wu. 1983. Neurogenetic analysis of potassium currents in *Drosophila:* Synergistic effects on neuromuscular transmission in double mutants. *Journal of Neurogenetics.* 1:17–28.

Ganetzky, B., and C.-F. Wu. 1985. Genes and membrane excitability in *Drosophila. Trends in Neuroscience.* 8:322–326.

Ganetzky, B., and C.-F. Wu. 1986. Neurogenetics of membrane excitability in *Drosophila. Annual Review of Genetics.* 20:13–45.

Gho, M., and B. Ganetzky. 1992. Analysis of repolarization of presynaptic motor terminals in *Drosophila* larvae using potassium channel-blocking drugs and mutations. *Journal of Experimental Biology.* 170:93–111.

Guy, H. R., S. R. Durell, J. Warmke, R. Drysdale, and B. Ganetzky. 1991. Similarities in amino acid sequences of *Drosophila eag* and cyclic nucleotide-gated channels. *Science.* 254:730.

Iverson, L. E., M. A. Tanouye, H. A. Lester, N. Davidson, and B. Rudy. 1988. A-type potassium channels expressed from *Shaker* locus cDNA. *Proceedings of the National Academy of Sciences, USA.* 85:5723–5727.

Jan, L. Y., and Y. N. Jan. 1976. Properties of the larval neuromuscular junction in *Drosophila melanogaster. Journal of Physiology.* 262:189–214.

Jan, Y. N., L. Y. Jan, and M. J. Dennis. 1977. Two mutations of synaptic transmission in *Drosophila. Proceedings of the Royal Society of London.* 198:87–108.

Kamb, A., L. E. Iverson, and M. A. Tanouye. 1987. Molecular characterization of *Shaker,* a *Drosophila* gene that encodes a potassium channel. *Cell.* 50:405–413.

Kaplan, W. D., and W. E. Trout, III. 1969. The behavior of four neurological mutants of *Drosophila. Genetics.* 61:399–409.

Kaupp, U. B. 1991. The cyclic nucleotide-gated channels of vertebrae photoreceptors and olfactory epithelium. *Trends in Neuroscience.* 14:150–157.

Knaus, H.-G., K. Folander, M. Garcia-Calvo, M. L. Garcia, G. J. Kaczorowski, M. Smith, and R. Swanson. 1994. Primary sequence and immunological characterization of β-subunit of high conductance Ca^{2+}-activated K^+ channel from smooth muscle. *Journal of Biological Chemistry.* 269:17274–17278.

Komatsu, A., S. Singh, P. Rathe, and C.-F. Wu. 1990. Mutational and gene-dosage analysis of calcium-activated potassium channels in *Drosophila:* correlation of microscopic and macroscopic currents. *Neuron.* 4:313–321.

McManus, O. B., L. M. H. Helms, L. Pallanck, B. Ganetzky, R. Swanson, and R. J. Leonard. 1995. Functional consequences of the heteromeric structure of high-conductance calcium-activated potassium channels. In press.

Pallanck, L., and B. Ganetzky. 1994. Cloning and characterization of human and mouse homologs of the *Drosophila* calcium-activated potassium channel gene. *Human Molecular Genetics.* 3:1239–1243.

Pongs, O., N. Kecskemethy, R. Muller, I. Krah-Jentgens, A. Baumann, H. H. Kiltz, I. Canal, S. Llamazares, and A. Ferrus. 1988. *Shaker* encodes a family of putative potassium channel proteins in the nervous system of *Drosophila. EMBO Journal.* 7:1087–1096.

Robertson, G. A., J. W. Warmke, and B. Ganetzky. 1993. Functional expression of the *Drosophila* EAG K^+ channel gene. *Biophysical Journal.* 64:340*a.* (Abstr.)

Rubin, G. 1988. *Drosophila* as an experimental organism. *Science.* 240:1453–1459.

Rudy, B. 1988. Diversity and ubiquity of K^+ channels. *Neuroscience.* 25:729–749.

Salkoff, L., K. Baker, A. Butler, M. Covarrubias, M. D. Pak, and A. Wei. 1992. An essential "set" of K^+ channels conserved in flies, mice and humans. *Trends in Neuroscience.* 15:161–166.

Schachtman, D. P., J. I. Schroeder, W. J. Lucas, J. A. Anderson, and R. F. Gaber. 1992. Expression of an inward-rectifying potassium channel by the *Arabidopsis* KAT1 cDNA. *Science.* 258:1654–1658.

Sentenac, H., N. Bonneaud, M. Minet, F. Lacroute, J.-M. Salmon, F. Gaymard, and C. Grignon. 1992. Cloning and expression in yeast of a plant potassium ion transport system. *Science.* 256:663–665.

Strong, M., K. G. Chandy, and G. Gutman. 1993. Molecular evolution of voltage-sensitive ion channel genes: on the origins of electrical excitability. *Molecular Biology and Evolution.* 10:221–242.

Tanouye, M. A., and R. J. Wyman. 1980. Motor outputs of giant nerve fiber in *Drosophila. Journal of Neurophysiology.* 44:405–421.

Temple, B. L., D. M. Papazian, T. L. Schwarz, Y. N. Jan, and L. Y. Jan. 1987. Sequence of a probable potassium channel component encoded at the *Shaker* locus of *Drosophila. Science.* 237:770–775.

Timpe, L. C., Y. N. Jan, and L. Y. Jan. 1988. Four cDNA clones from the *Sh* locus of *Drosophila* induce kinetically distinct A-type potassium currents in *Xenopus* oocytes. *Neuron.* 1:659–667.

Warmke, J., R. Drysdale, and B. Ganetzky. 1991. A distinct potassium channel polypeptide encoded by the *Drosophila eag* locus. *Science.* 252:1560–1562.

Warmke, J. W., and B. Ganetzky. 1994. A family of potassium channel genes related to *eag* in *Drosophila* and mammals. *Proceedings of the National Academy of Sciences, USA.* 91:3438–3442.

Wu, C.-F., and B. Ganetzky. 1992. Neurogenetic studies of ion channels in *Drosophila. In* Ion Channels. Vol. 3. T. Narahashi, editor. Plenum Publishing Corp., New York. 261–314.

Wu, C.-F., B. Ganetzky, Y. N. Jan, L. Y. Jan, and S. Benzer. 1978. A *Drosophila* mutant with a temperature-sensitive block in nerve conduction. *Proceedings of the National Academy of Sciences, USA.* 75:4057–4051.

Wu, C.-F., B. Ganetzky, A.-X. Liu, and F. Haugland. 1983. Mutations of two genes affect different components of potassium currents in *Drosophila. Science.* 220:1076–1078.

Zhong, Y., and C.-F. Wu. 1991. Alteration of four identified K^+ currents in *Drosophila* muscle by mutations of *eag. Science.* 252:1562–1564.

Potassium Channels at Nodes of Ranvier: A Role in Disease?

Bruce L Tempel and William F. Hopkins

Geriatric Research, Education and Clinical Center, Veterans Affairs Medical Center, Seattle, Washington 98108, and the Departments of Medicine and Pharmacology, University of Washington School of Medicine, Seattle, Washington 98195

*Kcna*1 and *Kcna*2, two closely related *Shaker*-like murine potassium (K^+) channels, are likely to have arisen by means of a chromosomal duplication event early in vertebrate evolution. Highly conserved through mammalian evolution, we wondered whether or not they are functionally redundant. Expression studies in *Xenopus* oocytes reveal a significant difference in the voltage sensitivity between the two channels, with the voltage sensitivity of coexpression mixtures depending on the relative expression ratios of the two channels. Knowing that these channels are localized at nodes of Ranvier in axons and synaptic terminals, we have developed a model which suggests that different ratios of expression may be related to the ability to support different action potential frequencies. If, as our data suggest, these channels are involved in repolarizing the axonal action potential or in modulating neurotransmitter release, it is easy to imagine how mutations in *Kcna*1 might underlie some aspects of the phenotype of the human disease, episodic ataxia (Browne, Gancher, Nutt, Brunt, Smith, Kramer, and Litt, 1994).

That voltage-gated ion channels are causally related to mammalian disease has been established for sodium, chloride, and calcium channels (each reviewed in other chapters of this volume). In contrast, potassium (K^+) channel mutants have been described primarily in *Drosophila*, which provided the first clones for voltage-gated (Jan and Jan, 1989; Warmke, Drysdale, and Ganetzky, 1991) and calcium-activated K^+ channels (Atkinson, Robertson, and Ganetzky, 1991). Only very recently has the first mammalian K^+ channel mutant—a human disease related to mutations in *Kcna*1—been described by Litt and co-workers (Browne et al., 1994).

We have asked how voltage-gated K^+ channels might be related to disease using both genetic and functional approaches in the mouse. The chromosomal locus for each of several K^+ channel genes have been identified in both mice and, by others, in human genomes (Fig. 1; Lock, Gilbert, Street, Migeon, Jenkins, Copeland, and Tempel, 1994). These locations are coincident with the regional localizations of certain neurological mutants, though to our knowledge, no causal connection has been established between a voltage-gated K^+ channel and any mouse mutant. Nonetheless, analysis of the structure, distribution, and physiological function of *Kcna*1 (mKv1.1) and *Kcna*2 (mKv1.2) may provide insight into possible role(s) these genes play in health and disease.

Chromosomal Locations and Evolutionary Implications

Fig. 1 shows a dendrogram of voltage-gated K^+ channel genes in which branch sites indicate the amino acid sequence relatedness between the channel genes. Individual genes within a subfamily (e.g., *Shaker*-like channels) are related at the 70% level, whereas different subfamilies (e.g., *Shaker* vs *Shal*) are only ~40% identical (Strong,

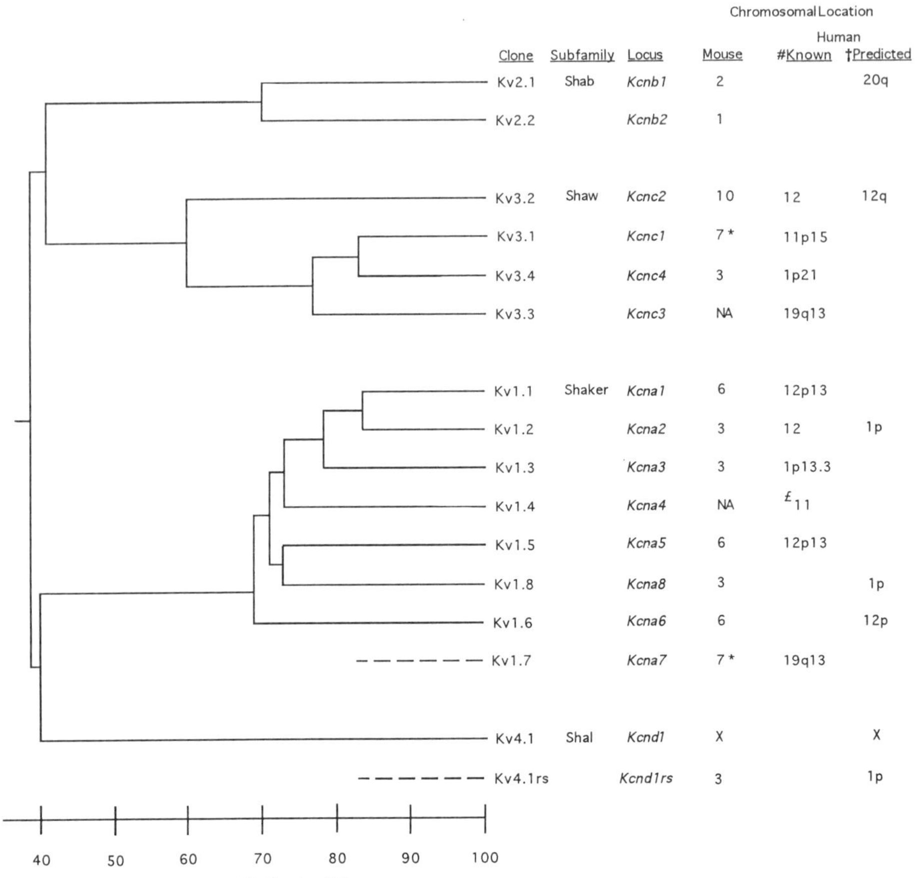

Figure 1. The voltage-gated potassium (K^+) channel gene family. Amino acid sequence alignment defines four different subfamilies: *Shaker, Shab, Shaw*, and *Shal*. The branch junctions approximate the values determined using the PileUp program for multigene alignments (GCG Package). Kv1.7 and Kv4.1rs could not be aligned due to lack of sequence information. NA = data not available. *These loci were determined in the same IB by K. G. Chandy and colleagues (Grissmer, Dethlefs, Wasmuth, Goldin, Gutman, Calahan, and Chandy, 1990. #Human chromosomal loci are summarized in Gutman and Chandy (1993). Our data from mouse is consistent with previous reports except for the localization of *KCNA2*, reported on human chromosome 12 (Grissmer et al., 1990) but predicted by our data to be within a cluster on 1p. Further, our data predicts that *KCNC2* is located on human 12q, refining the previous report that it localized to chromosome 12, but placing this gene outside the cluster on 12p. £Two locations have been reported for *KCNA4*: 11p14.1 (Gessler, Grupe, Grzeschik, and Pongs, 1992) and 11q13.4-q14.1 (Philipson, Eddy, Shows, and Bell, 1993). †These human loci are predicted from data in Lock et al. (1994).

Chandy, and Gutman, 1993; Lock et al., 1994). This discontinuity in sequence similarity corresponds to the functionally important ability of subunits within a subfamily to form functional heteromultimeric K^+ channels whereas subunits from different subfamilies appear to be excluded from forming heteromultimers (Isacoff, Jan, and Jan, 1990; Ruppersberg, Schroter, Sakmann, Stocker, Sewing, and Pongs, 1990; Covarrubias, Wei, and Salkoff, 1991). Also shown in Fig. 1 are the chromosomal locations of the genes. Notice that several genes are located on mouse

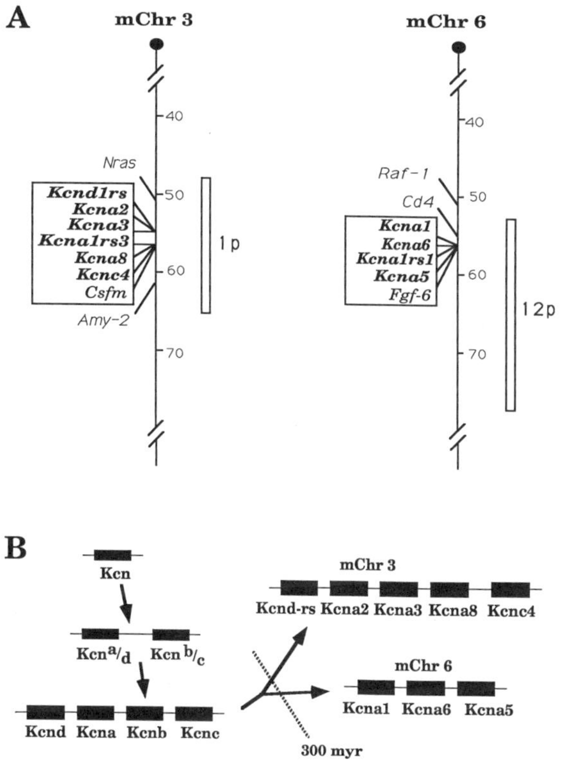

Figure 2. (*A*) Several K^+ channel genes exist in clusters on mouse chromosomes (mChr) 3 and 6. K^+ channel genes and adjacent loci are shown to the left of the chromosome. Homologous regions of human chromosomes (1p and 12p) are shown to the right of each mouse chromosome. (*B*) Schematic model depicting possible evolutionary events giving rise to the diversity of the voltage-gated K^+ channel gene family. An ancestral gene (K*cn*) is hypothesized to have duplicated, giving rise to two different genes: one that is hypothesized to have been the precursor ($Kcn^{a}/_{d}$) of the relatively closely related *Shaker* (*Kcna*) and *Shal* (*Kcnd*) subfamilies (Fig. 1); the other ($Kcn^{b}/_{c}$) being the precursor of the *Shab* (*Kcnb*) and *Shaw* (*Kcnc*) subfamilies. Local duplication of these two precursor genes, followed by sequence and functional divergence, is hypothesized to have established four different voltage-gated K^+ channel gene subfamilies sometime before the divergence of flies and mammals (>600 million years ago) (Tempel et al., 1988). Subsequent to the establishment of the K^+ channel subfamilies, chromosomal rearrangements are likely to have fragmented and dispersed the K channel genes to their modern locations. For example, a genome duplication event, hypothesized to have occurred ~ 300 million years ago, may be reflected in the K^+ channel clusters on mouse chromosomes 3 and 6. Modified from Lock et al. (1994).

chromosomes (mChr) 3 and 6. These K^+ channel gene loci were determined at relatively high resolution by analyzing the distribution of subspecies-specific restriction fragment length polymorphisms (RFLPs) in a panel of ~ 175 mice resulting from an interspecific backcross between *M.m. musculus* and *M.m. spretus* (Avner, Amar, Dandolo, and Guenet, 1988; Copeland and Jenkins, 1991). This analysis showed that at least five K^+ channel genes are clustered on mChr 3 while at least three additional genes are clustered on mChr 6 (Fig. 2*A*; Lock et al., 1994). Cloning of these regions in yeast artificial chromosomes has confirmed their physical proximity in the mouse genome (Migeon, Street, Demas, and Tempel, 1992; Street, V. A., and B. L. Tempel, manuscript in preparation).

The K^+ channel gene cluster on mChr 3 contains at least three members of the *Shaker*-like subfamily as well as one *Shaw*-like and one *Shal*-like gene. This clustering of distantly related K^+ channel genes suggests that the voltage gated K^+ channel gene family is likely to have arrisen from a series of local duplication events in ancestral time (Fig. 2 *B*; Lock et al., 1994). Because the same gene subfamilies are easily recognized in *Drosophila*, the sequences defining each subfamily must have diverged and been fixed over 600 million years ago (Tempel, Jan, and Jan, 1988). The fact that at least three *Shaker*-like genes are also clustered on mChr 6 means that these regions of mChr 3 and 6 are paralogous, perhaps having arisen by a genomic duplication event hypothesized to have occurred during the Devonian period, ~300 million years ago (Ohno, 1970). This hypothesis is supported by the existence of neurotrophic growth factor genes and *ras*-like oncogenes near the K^+ channel clusters on mChr 3 and 6, respectively (Lock et al., 1994).

The high level of amino acid sequence similarity between mKv1.1 on mChr 6 and mKv1.2 on mChr 3 also argues for their evolutionary relationship. Overall, these genes are 72% identical and within the transmembrane regions they are over 90% identical. This level of similarity brings up the question of whether Kv1.1 and Kv1.2 might not serve redundant functions in the nervous system. Arguing against redundancy we note that, for each gene, the sequence conservation between mouse and human channels is >99% overall, suggesting that their unique functions are important enough to have been conserved through mammalian evolution. In addition, Kv1.1 and Kv1.2 have overlapping but unique tissue distributions in the mouse brain and have significant physiological differences.

*Kcna*1 and *Kcna*2 Often Colocalize in Synaptic Regions, Dendrites and at Nodes of Ranvier in Axons

To study the distribution of *Kcna*1 and *Kcna*2 in the mouse brain, we developed antibody probes specific to each. Fusion proteins were produced from the relatively unique carboxyl-terminal regions of each K^+ channel and used to immunize rabbits. The resulting polyclonal seras were adsorption purified against the opposite fusion protein in order to remove cross-reacting antibodies. The resulting purified antisera proved to be highly specific, recognizing only the appropriate protein on immunoblots, in immunoprecipitation assays, and in immunohistochemical staining protocals (Wang, Kunkel, Martin, Schwartzkroin, and Tempel, 1993). Both channel proteins were found to be widely distributed in the brain, each occuring in specific dendrites, somata and synaptic-terminal regions of certain neurons (Sheng, Tsuar, Jan, and Jan, 1994; Wang, Kunkel, Schwartzkroin, and Tempel, 1994). In many instances *Kcna*1 and *Kcna*2 were colocalized to the same structures, for instance to the terminal plexus of basket cells in the cerebellum. In contrast, *Kcna*1 is expressed without detectable *Kcna*2 in CA3 pyramical cells and their axon collaterals in the hippocampal hilar region and *Kcna*2 is expressed in the absence of *Kcna*1 in olfactory mitral cells. A third localization pattern observed is one in which both channels are expressed in the same subcellular region, but their relative ratio of expression varies in different parts of the brain. For example, *Kcna*2 is localized to the middle molecular layer of the dentate gyrus, presumably in synaptic terminals of the perforant path which arises in the entorhinal cortex. *Kcna*1 is also localized to the middle molecular layer but in a gradient with stronger expression along the distal blades with little detectable expression near the apex of the dentate (Wang et al., 1994). Analogously, *Kcna*1 and *Kcna*2 are often colocalized to the juxtaparanodal regions of nodes of Ranvier on myelinated axons throughout the brain (Fig. 3). However, at some nodes, especially in smaller caliber axons, one channel or the other is seen to predominate in double-labeling experiments. These colocalization and differential expression patterns lead one to ask if heteromultimers of *Kcna*1 and *Kcna*2 form in vivo and if so, whether the heteromultimer has unique physiological properties.

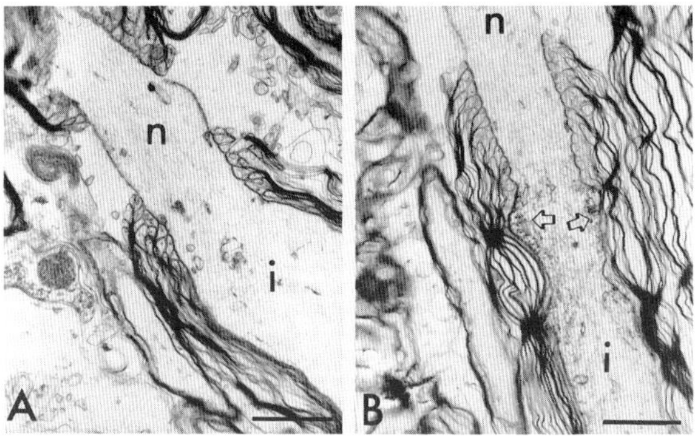

Figure 3. Electron micrographs of myelinated axons from mouse brain showing *Kcna*1 immunostaining. (*A*) Control axon in which primary antibody (a-*Kcna*1) was not added. (*B*) Axon showing localization of *Kcna*1 at juxtaparanodal region (*arrows*). Granular immunoreaction product is not seen at nodal (*n*) or internodal (*i*) membranes. EM immunocytochemistry as described in Wang et al. (1993).

*Kcna*1 and *Kcna*2 Form Heteromultimers with Intermediate Physiological Properties

Coimmunoprecipitation studies on solubilized mouse brain membranes have shown that *Kcna*1 and *Kcna*2 form heteromultimers in vivo (Wang et al., 1993). That other members of the *Shaker*-like, *Kcna* subfamily can heteromultimerize in vivo has been demonstrated for *Kcna*2 and *Kcna*4 (Sheng, Liao, Jan, and Jan, 1993) as well as for *Kcna*2 with *Kcna*1, *Kcna*4, and *Kcna*6 (Scott, Muniz, Sewing, Lichtinghagen, Parcej, Pongs, and Dolly, 1994). While these studies demonstrate that a fraction of various subtypes of the *Shaker*-like family of K^+ channels do heteromultimerize with other *Shaker*-like subunits, they do not prove that all *Shaker*-like subunits freely associate when coexpressed in the same cell. Subcompartmentalization of transcripts, isolated translation, or other forms of RNA or protein targeting may restrict the heteromultimerization of *Shaker*-like subunits.

To ask whether *Kcna*1 and *Kcna*2 can form heteromultimers in vitro and, if so, whether the heteromultimer has unique physiological properties, we have used the *Xenopus* oocyte expression system. When each of *Kcna*1 and *Kcna*2 is expressed alone, the resulting K^+ currents have very similar biophysical properties (Hopkins, Allen, Houamed, and Tempel, 1994). Both give rise to rapidly activating, sustained currents. Prepulse inactivation studies reveal that both have voltage-dependent, but incomplete, inactivation with *Kcna*2 showing greater inactivation. Onset and recovery from inactivation can be described by single, slow time constants for *Kcna*1 (2–4 s), while *Kcna*2 has a second, faster time constant (<400 ms). The voltage sensitivities for each are similar but the half-maximal voltages ($V_{1/2}$) differ by ~10 mV; *Kcna*2 being more positive than *Kcna*1 ($V_{1/2} = -37$ mV; Table I).

When *Kcna*1 and *Kcna*2 are coexpressed in *Xenopus* oocytes, they form heteromultimers (Christie, North, Osborne, Douglass, and Adelman, 1990; Hopkins et al., 1994). Allowing subunits to mix randomly, but changing the relative expression ratios between *Kcna*1 and *Kcna*2, we find that for most properties, the expression ratio determines the intermediate level of a particular biophysical property, for example, activation (Table I). Support for this conclusion has come from experiments in which

TABLE I
Summary of Biophysical Properties for mKv1.1, mKv1.2 and Heteromultimeric Channels Formed by Both

	Activation*			Prepulse inactivation‡		
	$V_{1/2}$	k	n	$V_{1/2}$	k	n
	mV			*mV*		
mKv1.1	−37 ± 2	6.1 ± 0.3	8	−49 ± 1	4.0 ± 0.3	5
mKv1.2	−27 ± 1	5.9 ± 0.2	16	−37 ± 1	4.5 ± 0.2	7
Coexpression ratio						
3 mKv1.2: 1 mKv1.1	−28 ± 1	7.2 ± 0.3	8	−39 ± 0.3	5.0 ± 0.2	7
1 mKv1.2: 2 mKv1.1	ND			−43 ± 0.6	5.0 ± 0.3	3
1 mKv1.2: 3 mKv1.1	−33 ± 1	5.9 ± 0.3	10	−48 ± 1	5.2 ± 0.3	8

*The voltage dependence of activation was assessed by obtaining K^+ current (I) − voltage (V) relations using 1-s voltage pulses from a holding potential of −70 mV and deriving conductance (G) values at each voltage with $G = I/(V - E_K)$ where E_K was measured in each oocyte as the K^+ tail current reversal potential. $G - V$ data were then fit with a Boltzmann equation: $G = G_{max}/(1 + \exp[V - V_{1/2}/k])$, where $V_{1/2}$ is the voltage at which G is half maximal and k is the increment in voltage required to alter the conductance by e-fold. (ND, not determined.)
‡Prepulse inactivation was determined as follows: from a holding potential of −70 mV, 5-s conditioning pulses were made to voltages between −90 and 10 mV followed by a 250-ms test pulse to 20 mV. Test pulse current was plotted as a function of conditioning pulse voltage and the data were fit with a modified Boltzmann equation: $I = (1 - F_s)/(1 + \exp[V - V_{1/2}/k]) + F_s$, where F_s refers to the noninactivating fraction of the total current.
Modified from Hopkins et al. (1994).

the subunit stoichiometry is constrained by using tandem cDNA constructs (Hurst, Kavanaugh, Yakel, Adelman, and North, 1992). One exception to the conclusion is that at all expression ratios the noninactivating fraction of the current was more similar to the value for *Kcna*1 than for *Kcna*2. The functional consequences, if any, for this dominant property of *Kcna*1 is not clear. Nonetheless, the result that expression ratio determines an intermediate $V_{1/2}$ may allow neurons expressing both channels to fine tune their physiological properties. This may be especially important in mammalian cells where the $V_{1/2}$ for *Kcna*1 is −24.9 ± 2.6 mV, whereas $V_{1/2}$ for *Kcna*2 is +23.4 ± 2.9 mV (Werkman, Kawamura, Yokoyama, Higashida, and Rogawski, 1992; Bosma, Allen, Martin, and Tempel, 1993).

*Kcna*1 and *Kcna*2 in a Model Cell

Except for their differences in half-maximal activation, the biophysical properties of *Kcna*1 and *Kcna*2 are quite similar. In an attempt to gain insight into the functional consequences of expression of *Kcna*1 and *Kcna*2, we developed a model of a neuron using Nodus 3.2 (DeSchutter, 1989) running on a Macintosh Quadra 900 computer. As a starting point, we chose a simple, one-compartment neuron in which to express the two potassium channel subtypes singly or together with a fast sodium conductance (Traub, 1982) and a small leakage conductance. The conductances were implemented with equations that closely followed Hodgkin-Huxley formalism (Hodgkin and Huxley, 1952). The equations that determine the voltage-dependent rate constants for the potassium conductances were determined by trial-and-error to yield conductance-voltage curves that closely matched the voltage dependence of activation obtained from the *Xenopus* oocyte expression data (Hopkins et al., 1994). Because the inactivation rates for *Kcna*1 and *Kcna*2 are both very slow, we simplified the model somewhat by making both conductances noninactivating to increase the speed of the simulations. The electrotonic parameters of the model cell, the equations that describe the voltage and time dependence of the conductances, and the conductance densities used in the model are given in the Appendix.

One way to assess the functional consequences of the expression of these potassium conductances is to quantitate their effects on the input-output characteristics of the model cell. To do this, we performed simulations in which constant current pulses of varying amplitudes were used to evoke action potential firing in the neuron, as if we had placed a microelectrode into it. We plotted the action potential firing frequency as a function of the amplitude of the current pulse. This approach has been used to characterize the firing properties of neurons and is commonly referred to as a frequency-current (*f-I*) curve. Fig. 4 *A* shows the results of a large number of simulations in which *Kcna*1 or *Kcna*2 are expressed singly or together as homomultimers. Two major conclusions emerge from these model results. First, although the biophysical properties of the potassium channels encoded by *Kcna*1 and *Kcna*2 are very similar, the *f-I* curves for the two are significantly different. Specifically, *Kcna*2 supports higher spike frequencies than *Kcna*1. Thus, a seemingly small 10-mV difference in the voltage dependence of activation can result in a significant change in the input-output characteristics of a model neuron. The larger 40-mV difference between $V_{1/2}$ values for *Kcna*1 and *Kcna*2 expressed in mammalian cells allows an even larger range of properties in the model neuron (data not shown). Second, when *Kcna*1 and *Kcna*2 are coexpressed as homomultimers in either a 1:1 or 1:2 ratio, respectively, the *f-I* curves are nearly identical to the *f-I* curve of *Kcna*1 alone. Thus, in spite of there being twice as many *Kcna*2 channels as *Kcna*1 channels in the model cell membrane, the *Kcna*1 spike firing phenotype dominates the *f-I* characteristic. This model result strongly suggests that one could not easily achieve an *f-I* curve that is intermediate or significantly different from *Kcna*1 or *Kcna*2 simply by coexpressing *Kcna*1 and *Kcna*2 homomultimeric channels in some ratio.

We next investigated the *f-I* curve in a model neuron in which *Kcna*1 and *Kcna*2 are allowed to form heteromultimers randomly. Based on previous experimental data (Hopkins et al., 1994), we modeled the effect of heteromultimer formation between *Kcna*1 and *Kcna*2 by using an intermediate conductance-voltage curve. The results of several simulations with these data are shown in Fig. 4 *B*. The *f-I* curve is clearly intermediate between the curves for *Kcna*1 and *Kcna*2 homomultimers. Therefore, the ability of *Kcna*1 and *Kcna*2 subunits to coassemble into heteromultimeric channels increases the dynamic range of spike frequencies in this model neuron in a manner that cannot easily be achieved by *Kcna*1 and *Kcna*2 homomultimers alone. This supports the intuitive notion that the increased molecular diversity afforded by heteromultimeric potassium channels is manifested as increased functional diversity in the electrical properties of a model neuron. Extrapolating to the situation in vivo, the model implies that differences in voltage responsiveness,

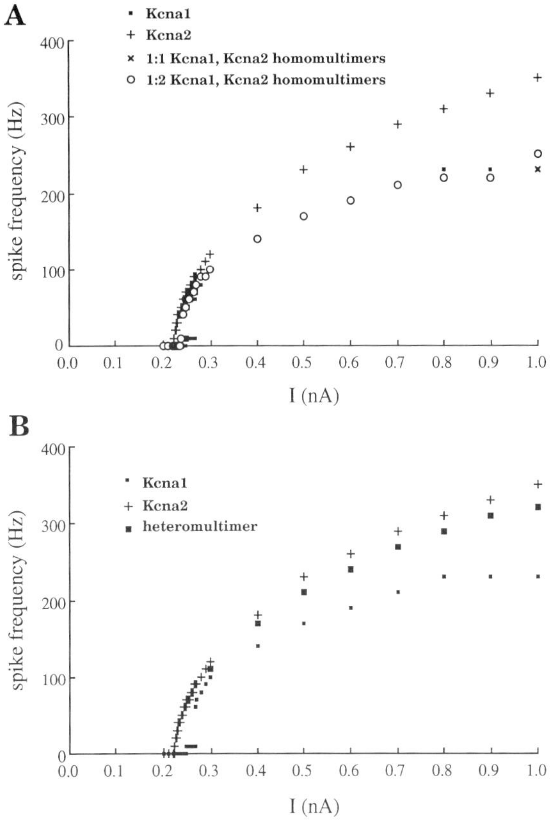

Figure 4. Current clamp simulations with a model neuron. (*a*) Frequency-current (*f-I*) curves for *Kcna*1, *Kcna*2, and for coexpression of two different ratios of the two types of potassium channel subunits as homomultimers. The data for *Kcna*1, and the two coexpression experiments are superimposed throughout most of the graph; (*b*) frequency-current (*f-I*) curves for *Kcna*1, *Kcna*2, and for coexpression of both as heteromultimers (see text for details).

whether naturally occurring between different *Shaker*-like subunits or induced by mutations in a particular subunit, can affect physiological function.

Potassium Channels in Disease

Chromosomal localization studies have shown that K^+ channel gene loci are sometimes coincident with regions that are known to contain mutant loci in mice or disease genes in humans. In mice, two neurological mutations, *opisthotonos* (*opt*) and *deafwaddler* (*dfw*), are found in the region of *Kcna1*, *Kcna5*, *Kcna6*, and *Kcna1rs1* on Chr 6. In humans, physiological syndromes associated with chromosomal regions containing K^+ channel genes include: (*a*) on 11p, long QT syndrome (Keating,

Atkinson, Dunn, Timothy, Vincent, and Leppert, 1991); (*b*) trisomy of chromosome 12p is associated with spike and wave discharges that underlie epileptic seizure activity (Guerrini, Bureau, Mattei, Battaglia, Galland, and Roger, 1990); (*c*) at 12q23–24, spinocerebellar ataxia (Gispert et al., 1993); and (*d*) on chromosome 20q, benign familial neonatal convulsions (Leppert, Anderson, Quattlebaum, Stauffer, O'Connell, Nakamura, Lalouel, and White, 1989). To date, none of these diseases have been shown to be causally related to mutations in any of the known K^+ channel genes. Further studies are needed to confirm or eliminate any relationship.

The first mammalian disease found to be associated with a K^+ channel is episodic ataxia/myokymia, a rare autosomal dominant disorder that causes brief episodes of ataxia induced by stress and rippling of the muscles between attacks (Browne et al., 1994). In each of four families with the disease, different point mutations were identified in KCNA1. In three out of four families, the mutation occurred in a transmembrane region, suggesting that the mutations may affect channel gating or voltage sensitivity. In light of our studies showing that relatively subtle changes in voltage sensitivity between *Kcna*1 and *Kcna*2 can significantly affect the input-output characteristics of a model neuron one can speculate that mutations affecting the voltage sensitivity of KCNA1 might have similar effects. Taking into account the complex tissue distribution of *Kcna*1, interpretation of the physiological changes occurring in patients with episodic ataxia/myokymia will require further study as well as the development of mouse models of this disease.

Appendix

The principal equation describing the change in intracellular potential $[V(t)]$ is

$$dV/dt = (I_{\text{input}} + I_{\text{Na}} + I_{\text{Kcnax}} + I_{\text{leak}})/C_{\text{n}},$$

where C_{n} is the total membrane capacitance, I_{input} equals the constant current stimulus pulse amplitude, and the ionic currents are defined as follows.

Fast Sodium Current

$$I_{\text{Na}} = G_{\text{Na}} m^3 h(V - E_{\text{Na}}).$$

Activation variable:

$$dm/dt = \alpha_{\text{m}} - (\alpha_{\text{m}} + \beta_{\text{m}})m$$

$$\alpha_{\text{m}} = (-18.24 - 0.32\,V)/-1.0 + e^{[(57+V)/-4]}\ \beta_{\text{m}} = (8.4 + 0.28V)/-1.0 + e^{[(30+V)/5]}.$$

Inactivation variable:

$$dh/dt = \alpha_{\text{h}} - (\alpha_{\text{h}} + \beta_{\text{h}})h$$

$$\alpha_{\text{h}} = 0.128/e^{[(53+V)/18]}\ \beta_{\text{h}} = 4/1.0 + e^{[(30+V)/-5]}.$$

Kcna1, Kcna2, Heteromultimer Potassium Current

$$I_{\text{Kcnax}} = G_{\text{Kcnax}} n^4\,(V - E_{\text{K}}).$$

Activation variable:

$$dn/dt = \alpha_{\text{n}} - (\alpha_{\text{n}} + \beta_{\text{n}})n.$$

*Kcna*1 rate constants:

$$\alpha_n = (-0.6 - 0.01\,V)/-1.0 + e^{[(60+V)/-3]}\ \beta_n = 0.4/e^{[(70+V)/13.5]}.$$

*Kcna*2 rate constants:

$$\alpha_n = (-0.6 - 0.01\,V)/-1.0 + e^{[(60+V)/-3]}\ \beta_n = 2.4/e^{[(70+V)/11]}.$$

Heteromultimer rate constants:

$$\alpha_n = (-0.6 - 0.01\,V)/-1.0 + e^{[(60+V)/-3]}\ \beta_n = 1.4/e^{[(70+V)/12.25]}.$$

Leakage Current

$$I_{leak} = G_{leak}(V - E_{leak}).$$

Model Parameters

Cell diameter, $d = 21\ \mu m$.
Total membrane capacitance, $C_n = 41.6$ pF.
Specific membrane capacitance, $C_m = 3.0\ \mu F\ cm^{-2}$.
Specific membrane resistance, $R_m = 10\ k\Omega\ cm^2$.
Specific cytoplasmic resistivity, $R_i = 100\ \Omega$ cm.
Resting potential, $V_{rest} = -70$ mV.
Sodium equilibrium potential, $E_{Na} = 45$ mV.
Potassium equilibrium potential, $E_K = -90$ mV.
Leakage equilibrium potential, $E_{leak} = -70$ mV.
Maximal sodium conductance, $G_{Na} = 50\ mS\ cm^{-2}$.
Maximal potassium conductance, $G_{Kcnax} = 200\ mS\ cm^{-2}$, where *Kcna*x can refer to *Kcna*l, *Kcna*2, some ratio of both together, or heteromultimers consisting of *Kcna*1 and *Kcna*2 subunits depending on the experiment.
Maximal leakage conductance $G_{leak} = 2\ mS\ cm^{-2}$.
See De Schutter (1989) for further modeling details.

References

Atkinson, N. S., G. A. Robertson, and B. Ganetzky. 1991. A component of calcium-activated potassium channels encoded by the *Drosophila slo* locus. *Science.* 253:551–555.

Avner, P., L. Amar, L. Dandolo, and J. L. Guenet. 1988. Genetic analysis of the mouse using interspecific crosses. *Trends in Genetics*. 4:18–23.

Bosma, M. M., M. L. Allen, T. M. Martin, and B. L Tempel. 1993. PKA-dependent regulation of mKv1.1, a mouse *Shaker*-like potassium channel gene, when stably expressed in CHO cells. *Journal of Neuroscience*. 13:5242–5250.

Browne, D. L., S. T. Gancher, J. G. Nutt, E. R. P. Brunt, E. A. Smith, P. Kramer, and M. Litt. 1994. Episodic ataxia/myokymia syndrome is associated with point mutations in the human potassium channel gene, *KCNA*1. *Nature Genetics.* 3:136–140.

Christie, M. J., R. A. North, P. B. Osborne, J. Douglass, and J. P. Adelman. 1990. Heteropolymeric potassium channels expressed in *Xenopus* oocytes from cloned subunits. *Neuron.* 4:405–411.

Copeland, N. G., and N. A. Jenkins. 1991. Development and applications of a molecular genetic linkage map of the mouse genome. *Trends in Genetics.* 7:113–118.

Covarrubias, M., A. Wei, and L. Salkoff. 1991. *Shaker, Shal, Shab*, and *Shaw* express independent K^+ current systems. *Neuron.* 7:763–773.

DeSchutter, E. 1989. Computer software for development of and simulation of compartmental models of neurons. *Computers in Biology and Medicine.* 19:71–81.

Gessler, M., A. Grupe, K. H. Grzeschik, and O. Pongs. 1992. The potassium channel HK1 maps to human chromosome 11p14.1 close to the FSHB gene. *Human Genetics.* 90:319–321.

Gispert, S. et al. 1993. Chromosomal assignment of the second locus for autosomal dominant cerebellar ataxia (SCA2) to chromosome 12q23–24.1. *Nature Genetics.* 4:295–299.

Grissmer, S., B. Dethlefs, J. J. Wasmuth, A. L. Goldin, G. A. Gutman, M. D. Cahalan, and K. G. Chandy. 1990. Expression and chromosomal localization of a lymphocyte K^+ channel gene. *Proceedings of the National Academy of Sciences, USA.* 87:9411–9415.

Guerrini, R., M. Bureau, M. G. Mattei, A. Battaglia, M. C. Galland, and J. Roger. 1990. Trisomy 12p syndrome: a chromosomal disorder associated with generalized 3-Hz spike and wave discharges. *Epilepsia.* 31:557–566.

Gutman, G. A., and K. G. Chandy. 1993. Nomenclature of mammalian voltage-dependent potassium channel genes. *Seminars in the Neurosciences.* 5:101–106.

Hodgkin, A. L., and A. F. Huxley. 1952. A quantitative description of membrane current and its application to conduction and excitation in nerve. *Journal of Physiology.* 117:500–544.

Hopkins, W. F., M. L. Allen, K. M. Houamed, and B. L Tempel. 1994. Properties of voltage-gated K^+ currents expressed in *Xenopus* oocytes by mKv1.1, mKv1.2 and their heteromultimers as revealed by mutagenesis of the dendrotoxin binding site in mKv1.1. *Pflügers Archiv.* 428:382–390.

Hurst, R. S., M. P. Kavanaugh, J. Yakel, J. P. Adelman, and R. A. North. 1992. Cooperative interactions among subunits of a voltage-dependent potassium channel. *Journal of Biological Chemistry.* 267:23742–23745.

Isacoff, E. Y., Y. N. Jan, and L. Y. Jan. 1990. Evidence for the formation of heteromultimeric potassium channels in *Xenopus* oocytes. *Nature.* 345:530–534.

Jan, L. Y., and Y. N. Jan. 1989. Voltage-sensitive ion channels. *Cell.* 56:13–25.

Keating, M., D. Atkinson, C. Dunn, K. Timothy, G. M. Vincent, and M. Leppert. 1991. Linkage of a cardiac arrhythmia, the Long QT syndrome, and the Harvey *ras-1* gene. *Science.* 252:704–706.

Leppert, M., V. E. Anderson, T. Quattlebaum, D. Stauffer, P. O'Connell, Y. Nakamura, J.-M. Lalouel, and R. White. 1989. Benign familial neonatal convulsions linked to genetic markers on chromosome 20. *Nature.* 337:647–648.

Lock, L. F., D. J. Gilbert, V. A. Street, M. B. Migeon, N. A. Jenkins, N. G. Copeland, and B. L Tempel. 1994. Voltage-gated potassium channel genes are clustered in paralogous regions of the mouse genome. *Genomics.* 20:354–362.

Migeon, M., V. A. Street, V. P. Demas, and B. L Tempel. 1992. Cloning, sequence and chromosomal localization of MK6, a murine potassium channel gene. *Epilepsy Research (Suppl.)* 9:173–181.

Ohno, S. 1970. Evolution by Gene Duplication. Springer-Verlag, New York.

Philipson, L. H., R. L. Eddy, T. B. Shows, and G. I. Bell. 1993. Assignment of human potassium channel gene *KCNA*4 (Kv1.4, PCN2) to chromosome 11q13.4—q14.1. *Genomics.* 15:463–464.

Ruppersberg, J. P., K. H. Schroter, B. Sakmann, M. Stocker, S. Sewing, and O. Pongs. 1990. Heteromultimeric channels formed by rat brain potassium-channel proteins. *Nature.* 345:535–537.

Scott, V. E. S., Z. M. Muniz, S. Sewing, R. Lichtinghagen, D. N. Parcej, O. Pongs, and J. O. Dolly. 1994. Antibodies specific for distinct Kv subunits unveil a heterooligomeric basis for subtypes of a-dendrotoxin-sensitive K^+ channels in bovine brain. *Biochemistry.* 33:11084–11088.

Sheng, M., Y. J. Liao, Y. N. Jan, and L. Y. Jan. 1993. Presynaptic A-current based on heteromultimeric K^+ channels detected *in vivo*. *Nature.* 365:72–75.

Sheng, M., M. L. Tsuar, Y. N. Jan, and L. Y. Jan. 1994. Contrasting subcellular localization of the Kv1.2 K^+ channel subunits in different neurons of rat brain. *Journal of Neuroscience.* 14:2408–2417.

Strong, M., K. G. Chandy, and G. A. Gutman. 1993. Molecular evolution of voltage-sensitive ion channel genes: on the origins of electrical excitability. *Molecular Biology and Evolution.* 10:221–242.

Tempel, B. L, Y. N. Jan, and L. Y. Jan. 1988. Cloning of a probable potassium channel gene from mouse brain. *Nature.* 332:837–839.

Traub, R. D. 1982. Simulation of intrinsic bursting in CA3 hippocampal neurons. *Neuroscience.* 7:1233–1242.

Wang, H., D. D. Kunkel, T. M. Martin, P. A. Schwartzkroin, and B. L Tempel. 1993. Heteromultimeric K^+ channels in terminal and juxtaparanodal regions of neurons. *Nature.* 365:75–79.

Wang, H., D. D. Kunkel, P. A. Schwartzkroin, and B. L Tempel. 1994. Localization of Kv1.1 and Kv1.2, two K channel proteins, to synaptic terminals, somata and dendrites in the mouse brain. *Journal of Neuroscience.* 14:4588–4599.

Warmke, J., R. Drysdale, and B. Ganetzky. 1991. A distinct potassium channel polypeptide encoded by the *Drosophila eag* locus. *Science.* 252:1560–1562.

Werkman, T. R., T. Kawamura, S. Yokoyama, H. Higashida, and M. A. Rogawski. 1992. Charybdotoxin, dendrotoxin, and mast cell degranulating peptide block the voltage-activated K^+ current of fibroblast cells stably transfected with NGK1 (Kv1.2) K^+ channel complimentary DNA. *Neuroscience.* 50:935–946.

Molecular Genetics of Long QT Syndrome

Mark T. Keating

Cardiology Division, Department of Human Genetics and the Eccles Program in Human Molecular Biology and Genetics, University of Utah, Salt Lake City, Utah 84112

In the long QT syndrome (LQT), individuals suffer from syncope, seizures and sudden death due to cardiac arrhythmias, specifically torsade de pointes and ventricular fibrillation. Many of these individuals also have prolongation of the QT interval on electrocardiograms, suggesting abnormal cardiac repolarization. To improve our understanding of the mechanisms underlying LQT and to facilitate presymptomatic diagnosis, we have begun to study families with autosomal dominant LQT. In 1991, we reported tight linkage between the LQT phenotype and the Harvey *ras*-1 gene (HRAS) in several families of Northern European descent. This discovery localized an LQT gene to chromosome 11p15.5 and made presymptomatic diagnosis in some families possible. In initial experiments, no recombination between HRAS and LQT was observed, making this protoncogene a candidate for LQT. This hypothesis was supported by physiologic data; other investigators had shown that ras proteins modulate cardiac potassium channels and an abnormality of potassium homeostasis could explain LQT. We eliminated HRAS as a candidate, however, by sequencing the coding region in 10 unrelated patients and finding no mutations. This indicated that the LQT locus was nearby, but not HRAS. Autosomal dominant LQT was previously thought to be genetically homogenous and the first seven LQT families we studied were linked to 11p15.5. In 1992, however, several groups, including my laboratory, identified locus heterogeneity for LQT. Recently we identified a second LQT locus, LQT2, on chromosome 7q35-36. Because several families were unlinked, at least one more LQT locus exists. This degree of heterogeneity presents opportunities. It seems likely, for example, that proteins encoded by distinct LQT genes interact to modulate cardiac repolarization. Identification and characterization of these genes may improve our understanding of repolarization-related arrhythmias.

Introduction

Long QT syndrome (LQT) is a cardiac disorder that causes syncope, seizures and sudden death (Vincent, Abildskov, and Burgess, 1974; Schwartz, Periti, and Malliani, 1975). Two forms of inherited LQT have been identified, autosomal dominant and autosomal recessive (Jervell and Lange-Nielsen, 1957; Romano, Gemme, and Pongiglione, 1963; Ward, 1964). Autosomal dominant LQT (also known as Romano-Ward syndrome), by far the most common form, has been found in all age and ethnic groups. Individuals affected by this disorder usually have a normal phenotype except for prolongation of the QT interval on surface electrocardiograms. The clinical features of LQT result from episodic cardiac arrhythmias specifically ventricular tachyarrhythmias like torsade de pointes and ventricular fibrillation. Although LQT is not a common diagnosis, repolarization-related arrhythmias are very common; more than 300,000 United States citizens die suddenly every year and in many cases the underlying mechanism is probably abnormal cardiac repolarization (Schwartz and Wolf, 1978; Kannel, Cupples, and D'Agostino, 1987; Willich, Levy, Rocco, Tofler, Stone, and Muller, 1987; Day, McComb, and Campbell, 1990; Meyerberg, Kessler, and Castellanos, 1993). LQT, therefore, provides an unprecedented opportunity to study life-threatening cardiac arrhythmias at the molecular level.

The First LQT Locus, LQT1, Was Mapped to Chromosome 11p15.5

After developing a phenotypic strategy for studying this disorder, my laboratory discovered tight linkage between autosomal dominant LQT and a polymorphism at HRAS 11. This discovery localized an LQT gene to chromosome 11p15.5 and made presymptomatic diagnosis possible in some families (Fig. 1). In initial experiments

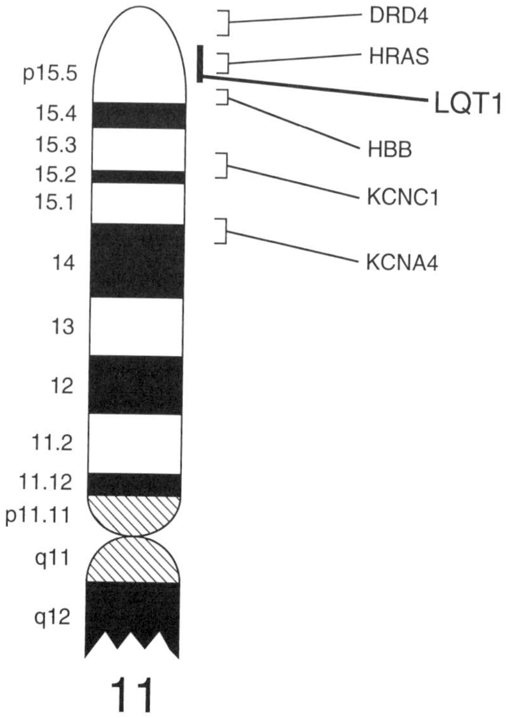

Figure 1. Ideogram and genetic map of chromosome 11 showing the location of LQT1.

we found no evidence of recombination between HRAS and LQT (Keating, Dunn, Atkinson, Timothy, Vincent, and Leppert, 1991*a;* Keating, Atkinson, Dunn, Timothy, Vincent, and Leppert, 1991*b*). This linkage made HRAS a candidate, a hypothesis supported by physiologic data. Other workers had shown that ras proteins modulate cardiac potassium channels and abnormalities of potassium homeostasis could explain LQT (Yatani et al., 1990). We eliminated HRAS as a candidate, however, by sequencing the coding region in 10 unrelated patients and finding no mutations. These data indicated that the LQT locus was nearby, but not HRAS.

Before these studies, autosomal dominant LQT was thought to be genetically homogenous, and the first 7 LQT families that we studied were linked to chromosome 11p15.5 (Keating et al., 1991*a,b*). In 1992, however, several laboratories, including my group, identified locus heterogeneity for LQT (Benhorin, Kalman, Madina, Towbin, Rave-Harel, Dyer, and Blangero, 1993; Keating, 1993; Curran, Atkinson, Timothy, Vincent, Moss, Leppert, and Keating, 1993; Towbin, Li, Taggart, Lehmann, Schwartz, Satler, Ayyagari, Robinson, Moss, and Hejtmancik, 1994). Thus, at least two LQT loci exist.

Phenotypic Analysis of Autosomal Dominant LQT

To identify LQT loci, we studied multigenerational families with autosomal dominant LQT. These families were not related; all were North Americans of varying descent including Polish, Italian, English, German, Swiss, Finnish, Norwegian, and Russian. Segregation analysis indicated an autosomal dominant pattern of LQT gene inheritance with incomplete penetrance in all families. These data suggested that some LQT gene carriers appeared unaffected. To avoid misclassifying individuals, we used the same conservative approach to phenotypic assignment that was

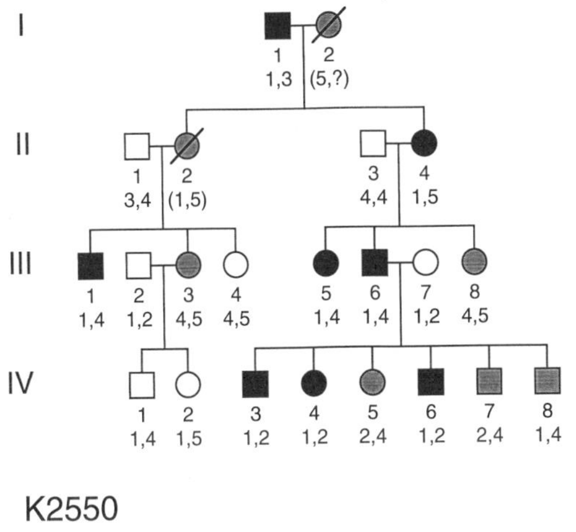

Figure 2. Pedigree structure in D7S483 genotypes for an autosomal dominant LQT family linked to chromosome 7. Affected individuals having the characteristic features of LQT (*circles*, females; squares, males). (*Empty circles or squares*) Unaffected individuals. Family members who had an equivocal phenotype or for whom no phenotypic data were available are stippled. Informed consent was obtained from all studied participants or their guardians in accordance with standards established by local institutional review boards.

successful in previous linkage studies (Keating et al., 1991*a,b;* Keating, 1992). Symptomatic individuals with a corrected QT interval (QTc) of 0.45 s or greater and asymptomatic individuals with a QTc of 0.45 s or greater were classified as affected. Asymptomatic individuals with a QTc of 0.41 s or less were classified as unaffected. Asymptomatic individuals with a QTc between 0.41 and 0.47 s and symptomatic individuals with a QTc of 0.41 s or less were classified as uncertain.

A Second LQT Locus, LQT2, Maps to Chromosome 7

We initiated linkage analysis in two families that are not linked to chromosome 11p15.5 (Curran et al., 1993). Genotypic analyses were performed with 110 STR markers that span the genome (Weber and May, 1989; Kramer, Becker, Heutink, James, Julier, Lathrop, Luty, Wang, Weber, Wilke, and Litt, 1992; Weissenbach, Gyapay, Dib, Vignal, Morissette, Millasseau, Vaysseix, and Lathrop, 1992; Gyapay, Morissette, Vignal, Dib, Fizames, Millasseau, Marc, Bernardi, Lathrop, and Weissenbach, 1994) including markers mapping near genes that were candidates based on a physiologic rationale. 70 markers were successfully scored and 35% of the genome

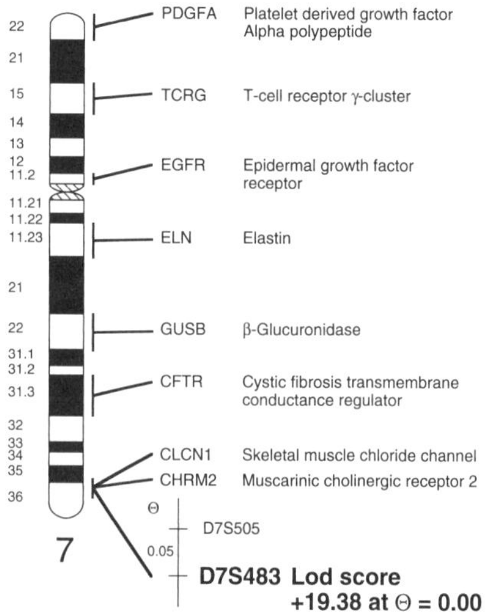

Figure 3. Ideogram of chromosome 7 showing approximate location of LQT2. The map shows sex-averaged recombination fractions between adjacent markers drawn to scale. The order and the distance are based on data from Genathon and the Human Genome-NIH-CEPH collaborative mapping group.

was excluded before linkage was identified. Evidence for linkage was identified using the marker D7S483 (Weissenbach et al., 1992; Gyapay et al., 1994). In one kindred the maximum lod score was 1.54 at a recombination fraction (q) of 0.001. The lod score for the second kindred was 2.71, also at $q = 0.001$. The combined lod scores for both families was 4.25 suggesting that a gene for LQT was located near D7S483 (Fig. 2).

To further test the hypothesis that a gene for LQT maps to the long arm of chromosome 7, we performed linkage analysis on 13 additional families. Seven families showed positive lod scores with D7S483. The lod score was greater than three in two families; the maximum combined lod score for nine families was 19.41. This score corresponds to odds favoring linkage of $> 10^{19}$. The maximum lod score was identified at a recombination fraction of $q = 0.001$, indicating that all affected individuals carry the disease allele. These data indicate tight linkage between D7S483 and a LQT disease gene (Fig. 3).

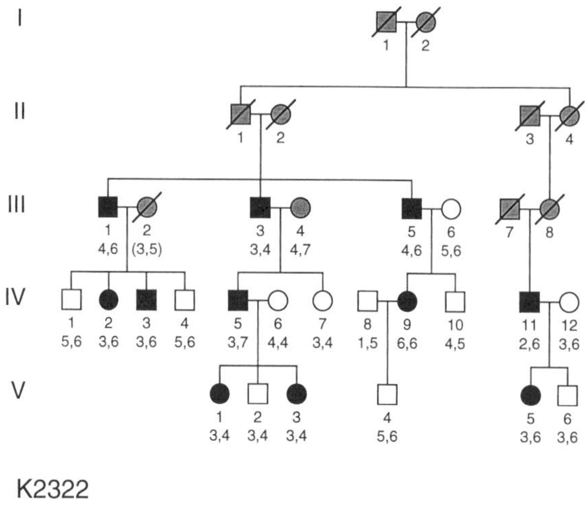

Figure 4. Pedigree structure for unlinked LQT families. Symbols are as described in the legend to Fig. 1.

Additional Locus Heterogeneity for LQT

The LQT phenotype was not linked to D7S483 in six families. Genotypic analysis with a neighboring polymorphic marker, D7S505 (Weissenbach et al., 1992; Gyapay et al., 1994) confirm the negative lod scores in all six families (Fig. 4). None of the 15 families demonstrated linkage to markers on chromosome 11p15.5. These data indicate that LQT is not linked to LQT1 or LQT2 in six families and that at least one more LQT locus exists.

Discussion

We have identified two loci for autosomal dominant LQT. The first locus designated LQT1, was mapped near HRAS on chromosome 11p15.5 in 1991 (Keating et al., 1991*a, b*). We recently used genetic linkage analysis to map a second LQT locus; designated LQT2, to chromosome 7q35-36. Two possible candidate genes for LQT2, a chloride channel (CLCN1) (George, Crackower, Abdalla, Hudson, and Ebers, 1993; Koch, Steinmeyer, Lorenz, Ricker, Wolf, Otto, Zoll, Lehmann-Horn, Grzeschik, and Jentsch, 1992) and a muscarinic receptor (CHRN2) (Bonner, Modi, Seuanez, and O'Brien, 1991; Goyal, 1989) have been mapped to this region. Reduced myocellular chloride currents could prolong action potential duration leading to secondary depolarizations in arrhythmia. Point mutations in CLCN1, which is expressed in skeletal and cardiac muscle are reported to cause Thompsen's disease, an inherited myotonia (George et al., 1993; Koch et al., 1992). Myotonia was not present in affected members of the families described here, but we have identified patients with both disorders, suggesting that they might have common mechanisms. A rationale for the involvement of muscarinic receptors in LQT can also be made; CHRN2 is primarily expressed in the heart and regulates cardiac-specific ion channels, particularly potassium channels (Bonner, Buckley, Young, and Brann, 1987; Bonner et al., 1991; Goyal, 1989). Mutations in these receptors might affect cardiac repolarization and increase the susceptibility of ventricular tachyarrhythmias. Refined linkage and mutational analyses will determine if either gene causes LQT.

The relative importance of the three or more LQT loci is not yet known. We have mapped 10 families to LQT1, nine families to LQT2 and six families remain unlinked. Examination of additional LQT families will help determine the relative importance of the different LQT loci. New linkage studies will define a third LQT locus; once it has been identified, we will determine if additional heterogeneity exists.

We conclude that two major genes predisposing individuals to cardiac arrhythmias are located on chromosomes 11 and 7 and that at least one more autosomal dominant LQT gene exists. The phenotypes of patients with these different forms of LQT are surprisingly similar. With the benefit of these genetic data we may now find subtle phenotypic differences between the different forms of LQT. It seems likely, however, that the repolarization abnormalities underlying different forms of LQT are the same. LQT genes, therefore, may encode elements of a common physiologic mechanism of arrhythmia. If so, characterization of this mechanism may simplify efforts to improve prediction, prevention and treatment of cardiac arrhythmias.

Methods

Clinical Analysis

Kindreds were ascertained through medical clinics across North America. Informed consent was obtained from all participants or their guardians in accordance with standards established by local institutional review boards. We obtained historical data and electrocardiograms from each family member and evaluated for the presence of syncope, syncopal episodes, the presence of seizures, the age of onset of symptoms and the occurrence of sudden death. Symptoms such as palpitations and light headedness were not included in the study.

Genotypic Analysis

Typing of PCR markers was performed as described by Weber and May with the following modifications (Weber and May, 1989). PCR was carried out with 50 ng DNA in a final volume of 10 ml using a Perkin-Elmer Cetus 9600 thermocycler. Amplification conditions were 94°C for 5 min followed by five cycles at 94°C for 10 s, X°C for 20 s, 72°C for 20 s, then 25 cycles of 94°C for 10 s, Y°C for 20 s, 72°C for 20 s. The aneeling temperatures, *X* and *Y* varied with the markers used (Weber and May, 1989; Kramer et al., 1992; Weissenbach et al., 1992; Gyapay et al., 1994). Ten ml of formamide loading dye was added to each reaction, samples were denatured to 94°C for 10 min and held on ice. Two ml of each sample were separated by electrophoresis on 6% denaturing polyacryamide gels which were drawn and exposed to x-ray film overnight at −70°C.

Linkage Analysis

To avoid bias, all polymorphisms were scored without knowledge of phenotypic data. The LINKAGE V5.1 software package was used to perform pairwise linkage analysis (Lathrop, Lalouel, Julier, and Ott, 1985). Penetrance was set at 0.90 and the LQT gene frequency was assumed to be 0.001 based on previous estimates. Recombination frequencies were assumed to be equal between males and females. Microsatellite alleles frequencies were assumed to be equal.

Acknowledgements

The molecular genetic work described in this manuscript was performed in my laboratory by Changan Jiang, Mark Curran, Igor Splawski, Donald Atkinson and Qing Wang. Ascertainment and phenotyping of LQT families and patients was completed in collaboration with Katherine Timothy, G. Michael Vincent, Arthur Moss, Peter Schwartz, Michael Lehmann, Tom Taggart, and Jeffrey Towbin.

This work was supported by National Institutes of Health Grant RO1HL48074 and the American Heart Association.

References

Benhorin, J., Y. Kalman, A. Madina, J. Towbin, N. Rave-Harel, T. D. Dyer, and J. Blangero. 1993. Evidence of genetic heterogeneity in the long QT syndrome. *Science.* 260:1960–1962.

Bonner, T., W. Modi, H. Seuanez, and S. O'Brien. 1991. Chromosomal mapping of five human genes encoding muscarine acetylcholine receptors. *Cytogenetic and Cell Genetics.* 58:1850–1867.

Bonner, T. I., N. J. Buckley, A. C. Young, and M. R. Brann. 1987. Identification of a family of muscarine acetylcholine receptor genes. *Science.* 237:527–532.

Curran, M., D. Atkinson, K. Timothy, G. M. Vincent, A. Moss, M. Leppert, and M. Keating. 1993. Locus heterogeneity of autosomal dominant long QT syndrome. *Journal of Clinical Investigation.* 92:799–803.

Day, C. P., J. M. McComb, and R. W. F. Campbell. 1990. QT dispersion: an indication of arrhythmia risk in patients with long QT intervals. *British Heart Journal.* 63:342–344.

George, A., M. Crackower, J. Abdalla, A. Hudson, and G. Ebers. 1993. Molecular basis of Thomsen's disease (autosomal dominant myotonia congenita). *Nature Genetics.* 3:305–309.

Goyal, R. 1989. Muscarine receptor subtypes. 1989. *The New England Journal of Medicine.* 321:1022–1029.

Gyapay, C., J. Morissette, A. Vignal, C. Dib, C. Fizames, P. Millasseau, S. Marc, G. Bernardi, M. Lathrop, and J. Weissenbach. 1994. The 1993–93 Genethon human genetic linkage map. *Nature Genetics.* 7:246–339.

Jervell, A., and F. Lange-Nielsen. 1957. Congenital deaf mutism, functional heart disease with prolongation of the QT interval and sudden death. *American Heart Journal.* 54:59–78.

Kannel, W. B., A. Cupples, and R. B. D'Agostino. 1987. Sudden death risk in overt coronary heart diseases: the Framingham study. *American Heart Journal.* 113:799–804.

Keating, M. 1993. Evidence for genetic heterogeneity in the long QT syndrome. *Science.* 260:960–1962.

Keating, M., C. Dunn, D. Atkinson, K. Timothy, G. M. Vincent, and M. Leppert. 1991*a*. Linkage of a cardiac arrhythmia, the long QT syndrome, and the Harvey *ras*-1 gene. *Science.* 252:704–706.

Keating, M., D. Atkinson, C. Dunn, K. Timothy, G. M. Vincent, and M. Leppert. 1991*b*. Linkage of the long QT syndrome to the Harvey ras-1 locus on chromosome 11. *American Journal of Human Genetics.* 49:1335–1339.

Keating, M. 1992. Linkage analysis of the long QT syndrome, using genetics to study cardiovascular disease. *Circulation.* 85:1973–1986.

Koch, M. C., K. Steinmeyer, C. Lorenz, K. Ricker, F. Wolf, M. Otto, B. Zoll, F. Lehmann-Horn, K-H. Grzeschik, and T. J. Jentsch. 1992. The skeletal muscle chloride channel in dominant and recessive human myotonia. *Science.* 257:797–800.

Kramer, P., W. Becker, P. Heutink, M. James, C. Julier, M. Lathrop, J. A. Luty, Z. Wang, J. L. Weber, P. Wilkie, and M. Litt. 1992. A comprehensive genetic linkage map of the Human Genome/NIH/CEPH collaborative Mapping Group. *Science.* 258:67–86.

Lathrop, G., J. Lalouel, C. Julier, and J. Ott. 1985. Multilocus linkage analysis in humans: detection of linkage and estimation of recombination. *American Journal of Human Genetics.* 37:482–498.

Myerburg, R. J., K. M. Kessler, and A. Castellanos. 1993. Sudden cardiac death: epidemiology, transient risk and intervention assessment. *Annals of Internal Medicine.* 119:1187–1197.

Romano, C., G. Gemme, and R. Pongiglione. 1963. Aritmie cardiache rare dell'eta'pediatrica. II. Accessi sincopali per fibrillazione ventricolare parossistica. *Clinical Pediatrics (Bologne).* 45:656–683.

Schwartz, P. J., M. Periti, and A. Malliani. 1975. The long QT syndrome. *American Heart Journal.* 89:378–390.

Schwartz, P. J., and S. Wolf. 1978. QT interval prolongation as predictor of sudden death in patients with myocardial infarction. *Circulation.* 57:1074–1077.

Towbin, J. A., H. Li, R. T. Taggart, M. Lehmann, P. Schwartz, C. Satler, R. Ayyagari, J. Robinson, A. Moss, and J. F. Hejtmancik. 1994. Evidence of genetic heterogeneity in Romano-Ward long QT syndrome (LQTS): analysis of 23 families. *Circulation.* 90:2635–2644.

Vincent, G. M., J. A. Abildskov, and M. J. Burgess. 1974. Q-T interval syndromes. *Progress in Cardiovascular Disease.* 16:523–530.

Ward, O. C. 1964. New familial cardiac syndrome in children. *Journal of Irish Medical Association.* 54:103–106.

Weber, J. L., and P. E. May. 1989. Abundant class of human DNA polymorphisms which can be typed using the polymerase chain reaction. *American Journal of Human Genetics.* 44:388–396.

Weissenbach, J., G. Gyapay, C. Dib, A. Vignal, J. Morissette, P. Millasseau, G. Vaysseix, and M. Lathrop. 1992. A second-generation linkage map of the human genome. *Nature.* 359:794–801.

Willich, S. N., D. Levy, M. Rocco, G. Tofler, P. H. Stone, and J. E. Muller. 1987. Circadian variation in the incidence of sudden cardiac death in Framingham heart study population. *American Journal of Cardiology.* 60:801–806.

Yatani, A., K. Okabe, P. Polakis, R. Halenbeck, F. McCormick, and A. M. Brown. 1990. Ras p21 and GAP inhibit coupling of muscrinic receptors to artial potassium channels. *Cell.* 61:769–776.

Chapter 3

Sodium Channel Disorders

Sodium Channel Mutations and Disorders of Excitation in Human Skeletal Muscle

Sen Ji,* Alfred L. George,[§] Richard Horn,[‡] and Robert L. Barchi*

**Departments of Neurology and Neuroscience and the Mahoney Institute of Neurological Sciences, University of Pennsylvania School of Medicine, Philadelphia, Pennsylvania 19104; [‡]Department of Physiology, Thomas Jefferson University School of Medicine Philadelphia, Pennsylvania 19107; and [§]Department of Medicine, Vanderbilt University School of Medicine, Nashville, Tennessee 37232*

Introduction

Because the voltage-dependent sodium channel in skeletal muscle sarcolemma generates the action potential necessary to link signals at the neuromuscular junction to activation of the contractile apparatus, it is not surprising that defects in this key membrane protein might cause human muscle disease (Barchi, 1994). Without this action potential, muscle paralysis will occur in spite of normal motor nerve, neuromuscular junction, and contractile protein function. If the sarcolemma produces multiple action potentials in response to a stimulus, a delay in muscle relaxation called myotonia can result, again interfering with function.

In the past few years, as our knowledge of the molecular aspects of sodium channels has grown, a number of diseases affecting muscle membrane excitability in humans have been linked to mutations in the gene encoding this channel in skeletal muscle (Barchi, 1993; Rüdel, Ricker, and Lehmann-Horn, 1993). While discovery of these mutations has provided valuable insight into the pathophysiology of these diseases, the mutations have also given us unexpected clues about the function of the normal channel.

The Periodic Paralyses

The periodic paralyses are a group of human muscle diseases characterized by episodes of skeletal muscle weakness or paralysis often occurring on the background of normal interictal strength. The most common forms are genetically determined and are inherited as an autosomal dominant trait. Affected individuals usually have no abnormalities of nerve or neuromuscular transmission. Although some develop permanent weakness with time, many appear completely normal on routine examination between bouts of paralysis (Barchi, 1993; Rüdel and Lehmann-Horn, 1985).

Clinicians have long been aware that the serum potassium concentration can change dramatically during an episode of periodic paralysis, and the direction of the shift is usually the same for all affected members of a kindred (Riggs, 1988). Based on these electrolyte shifts, families have been classified as having either hyperkalemic periodic paralysis (HyPP) or hypokalemic periodic paralysis (HoPP). While there is considerable overlap in symptoms, these two forms of periodic paralysis tend to differ in regard to the length, severity and frequency of their attacks (Table I). Of particular interest, HyPP patients often show evidence of myotonia, a form of muscle membrane hyperexcitability, while the HoPP families do not.

A third rare disorder, paramyotonia congenita (PC) (Streib, 1991), is usually grouped clinically with the periodic paralyses. Although individuals with PC show mostly signs of hyperexcitable muscle membranes, with myotonia and muscle stiffness brought on especially by cold exposure, they also have occasional episodes of paralysis. The myotonia in PC differs from that seen in the more common myotonia congenita, which is caused by a defect in the muscle chloride channel (Koch, Steinmeyer, Lorenz, Ricker, Wolf, Otto, Zoll, Lehmann-Horn, Grzeschik, and Jentsch, 1992), in growing worse with exercise (paradoxical myotonia) instead of being relieved by it.

Kindreds have been reported with what appears clinically to be classical myotonia; that is, myotonia that decreases in severity with exercise as it does in myotonia congenita. These families received particular attention either because of a

TABLE I
The Hereditary Periodic Paralyses

	Hypokalemic periodic paralysis	Hyperkalemic periodic paralysis	Paramyotonia congenita
Age of onset	Second decade	First decade	Birth
Attack frequency	Infrequent	Frequent	Rare
Attack severity	Severe	Moderate	Variable
Attack duration	Hours to days	Minutes to hours	Hours
Triggering factors	Rest after exercise	Rest after exercise	Cold
	Carbohydrate load	Hunger	Exercise
	Cold or stress	Cold	
Serum K^+	Low	High	Normal
Myotonia	None	Occasional	Prominent
Inheritance	Dominant	Dominant	Dominant

fluctuation in the severity of their symptoms or because of associated atypical features such as painful contractions or response to particular medications. Some of these families have also proven to be associated with sodium channel mutations rather than the expected defects in the muscle membrane chloride channel (Ptàček, Tawil, Griggs, Storvick, and Leppert, 1992*b*).

Muscle fibers in patients with PC or HyPP depolarize during a paralytic attack as the result of an increase in membrane conductance to sodium ions (Lehmann-Horn, Küther, Ricker, Grafe, Ballanyi, and Rüdel, 1987*a;* Lehmann-Horn, Rüdel, Ricker, Lorkovic, Dengler, and Hopf, 1983; Lehmann-Horn, Rüdel, and Ricker, 1987*b*). This persistent depolarization leads to inactivation of normal voltage-dependent sodium channels and failure of action potential propagation. The first real clue to the molecular pathophysiology of these diseases came with the demonstration that, in PC and HyPP fibers but not in HoPP muscle, this depolarization and its associated sodium current could be blocked by tetrodotoxin (TTX), directly implicating the voltage-dependent sodium channel in their pathogenesis (Lehmann-

Horn et al., 1983; Lehmann-Horn et al., 1987*a,b*). Subsequent electrophysiological studies demonstrated a small but persistent noninactivating component of the sodium current in voltage-clamped muscle fibers from patients with HyPP. More recent patch clamp measurements on cultured human myotubes grown from HyPP muscle biopsies have confirmed abnormalities of sodium channel function, with some channels showing repeated prolonged openings during a single depolarization, suggesting an abnormality in the inactivation process (Cannon, Brown, and Corey, 1991). Further progress in defining the role of sodium channels in these diseases, however, awaited the molecular characterization of the channel protein itself.

Muscle Sodium Channels

Voltage-dependent sodium channels in skeletal muscle resemble those in nerve and heart in having one large glycoprotein α subunit of ~260 kD which provides most of the primary channel functions. In mammalian skeletal muscle, a smaller β subunit (~38 kD) is also present in 1:1 stoichiometry with α (Barchi, 1988). While not necessary to the formation of a functional channel, β modifies the kinetic properties of α (Isom, De Jongh, Patton, Reber, Offord, Charbonneau, Walsh, Goldin, and Catterall, 1992).

Skeletal muscle expresses two sodium channel isoforms at different times in development and under different conditions of innervation (Kallen, Sheng, Yang, Chen, Rogart, and Barchi, 1990; Trimmer, Cooperman, Tomiko, Zhou, Crean, Boyle, Kallen, Sheng, Barchi, Sigworth, Goodman, Agnew, and Mandel, 1989; Yang, Sladky, Kallen, and Barchi, 1991). The α subunits of both forms have been cloned and characterized from rat and human muscle (Kallen et al., 1990; George, Komisarof, Kallen, and Barchi, 1991*a*). These sequences show features characteristic of this family of voltage-gated ion channels, with four large internal repeat domains, each containing six putative transmembrane segments. The fourth helix in each domain has the repeating motif of ($[R/K\text{-}X\text{-}X]_n$) which is the hallmark of these voltage-gated channels (Jan and Jan, 1989). The single β subunit in skeletal muscle has also been characterized; it is identical in sequence to that found in brain. Indeed, in humans, a single gene appears to encode the β subunit expressed in brain, heart and skeletal muscle (Makita, Bennett, and George, 1994).

For the principal adult skeletal muscle sodium channel isoform, SkM1, which is sensitive to tetrodotoxin, expression of the α subunit alone in oocytes produces channels with abnormally slow inactivation kinetics. There are two components in the current inactivation, each associated with a unique channel gating mode (Zhou, Potts, Trimmer, Agnew, and Sigworth, 1991). Individual channels can switch between these two gating modes, and the distribution of channels between modes is a function of membrane potential (Ji, Sun, George, Horn, and Barchi, 1994). Coexpression of the β subunit with α results in the stabilization of the channel conformation associated with the rapidly inactivating kinetic mode; this is the mode that predominates in vivo (Isom et al., 1992; Ji et al., 1994).

Using the cloned cDNA as a probe, the location and organization of the gene encoding the skeletal muscle sodium channel has been analyzed. The coding region of the channel gene, located at 17q23.1-25.3 (George, Ledbetter, Kallen, and Barchi, 1991*b*), contains 24 exons and 23 introns within a total of 34.5 kb of DNA (George, Iyer, Kleinfield, Kallen, and Barchi, 1993). Intron/exon junctions do not fall at points that divide functional or structural units, but the locations of these junctions are identical in the rat and human channel. The location and characterization of the SCN4A gene has provided the tools needed to evaluate the role of sodium channels in the hereditary periodic paralyses.

Sodium Channels and Periodic Paralysis

Using probes to the newly identified SCN4A locus, genetic linkage was demonstrated between this locus and the phenotypic expression of both PC and HyPP by several groups (Ebers, George, Barchi, Ting-Passador, Kallen, Lathrop, Beckmann, Hahn, Brown, Campbell, and Hudson, 1991; Fontaine, Khurana, Hoffman, Bruns, Haines, Trofatter, Hanson, Rich, McFarlane, Yesek, Romano, Guesella, and Brown, 1990; Koch, Ricker, Otto, Grimm, Hoffman, Rüdel, Bender, Zoll, Harper, and Lehmann-Horn, 1991. Ptàček, Trimmer, Agnew, Roberts, Petajan, and Leppert, 1991*b;* Ptàček, Tyler, Trimmer, Agnew, and Leppert, 1991*c*). Linkage with the gene for this channel

TABLE II
Sodium Channel Mutations Producing Human Muscle Disease

Genotype	Substitution	Region	Exon	Phenotype	Reference
C2188T	T704M	D2-S5	13	HYPP	Ptáček et al., 1991*a*
C2411T	S804F	D2-S6	14	SCM	McClatchey et al., 1992
G3466A	A1156T	D3-S4-5	19	HYPP/PC	McClatchey et al., 1992
A3555G	I1160V	D3-S4-5	19	SCM	Ptáček et al., 1994
G3917T	G1306V	D3-D4	22	SCM	McClatchey et al., 1992
G3917A	G1306E	D3-D4	22	SCM	Lerche et al., 1993
G3917C	G1306A	D3-D4	22	SCM	Lerche et al., 1993
C3938T	T1313M	D3-D4	22	PC	McClatchey et al., 1992
A4078G	M1360V	D4-S1	23	HYPP	Lehmann-Horn et al., 1993
T498G	L1433R	D4-S3	24	PC	Ptáček et al., 1993
C4342T	R1448C	D4-S4	24	PC	Ptáček et al., 1992
C4343A	R1448H	D4-S4	24	PC	Ptáček et al., 1992
G4765A	V1589M	D4-S6	24	SCM	Heine et al., 1993
A4774G	M1592V	D4-S6	24	HYPP	Rojas et al., 1991

isoform was also found in several families expressing unusual forms of what appeared otherwise to be myotonia congenita, suggesting a varied range of phenotypes for sodium channel mutations.

With the sequence of all exon/intron junctions in hand, families whose disease expression was linked to the *SCN4A* locus could be screened for gene mutations by amplification of these coding regions using PAR. The PAR products were then analyzed with techniques such as single strand conformational polymorphism (SSCP) and denaturing gradient gel electrophoresis (DGGE) that are capable of detecting single base differences in DNA segments of 500 bp or more in length. To date, 16 different point mutations have been reported; in each case, the identified mutation cosegregates with the disease phenotype, and is never seen as a random polymorphism in controls. These mutations are not evenly distributed throughout the channel primary sequence, but are concentrated in domains 2, 3, and 4, as well as in the ID3-4 linker. No mutations have been found in domain 1 (Table II).

Mutations in families with the HyPP phenotype are located in domains 2–4 either near the predicted cytoplasmic end of transmembrane helices or in the short cytoplasmic loops joining two helices. Mutations with the distinctive PC phenotype are found either in the ID3-4 linker or, surprisingly, at the extracellular end of D4-S4 and the adjacent S3 helix. Patients with the atypical myotonia phenotypes have mutations either in the ID3-4 linker or near the cytoplasmic ends of helices in domain 3 or 4.

Biophysical Studies of Periodic Paralysis Mutations

Although sodium channel mutations can be linked to disease through genetic analyses of kindreds, proof of a causal relationship between a particular mutation and the disease phenotype requires reconstruction and analysis of that mutation in the normal channel background. With full-length clones available for expression of the SkM1 channel, these experiments become feasible.

Mutations producing HyPP have been examined in the rat SkM1 channel by several groups (Cummins, Zhou, Sigworth, Ukomadu, Stephan, Ptàček, and Agnew, 1993; Cannon and Stritmatter, 1993). While the details emphasized by different groups have varied, several common features are evident. The T704M mutation, one of the most commonly encountered in HyPP kindreds, does not affect the kinetics of channel inactivation or recovery from inactivation. It does, however, produce small but significant shifts in the voltage dependence of both channel activation and inactivation, resulting in increased overlap of these curves. This overlap can lead to window currents in the voltage range at which mutant channels can remain open without inactivating (Cummins et al., 1993; Yang, Ji, Zhou, Ptáček, Barchi, Horn, and George, 1994). In addition, the mutation alters modal gating, causing an increase in the appearance of the slowly inactivating mode (Cannon and Strittmatter, 1993). These two alterations may account for the small noninactivating currents seen in HyPP muscle.

Effects of PC Mutations on hSkM1 Channel Gating

We have recently focused our studies on the mutations that produce the PC phenotype by constructing five PC mutations in hSkM1: A1156T (McClatchey, McKenna-Yasek, Cros, Worthen, Kuncl, De Silva, Cornblath, Gusella, and Brown, 1992), T1313M (McClatchey, Van den Bergh, Pericak-Vance, Raskind, Verellen, McKenna-Yasek, Rao, Haines, Bird, Brown, and Gusella, 1992*b*), L1433R (Ptáček, Gouw, Kwiecinski, McManis, Mendell, Barohn, George, Barchi, Robertson, and Leppert, 1993), R1448C and R1448H (Ptàček, George, Barchi, Griggs, Riggs, Robertson, and Leppert, 1992*a*). We compared the gating properties of these mutants with the wild-type hSkM1 sodium channel by examining currents in tsA 201 cells transiently transfected with each construct. According to a general model of sodium channel structure (Noda, Ikeda, Kayano, Suzuki, Takeshima, Kurasaki, Takahashi, and Numa, 1986), A1156T is in the S4-S5 cytoplasmic linker in D3; T1313M lies in the ID3-4 interdomain region; and L1433R and R1448C/H are at the extracellular ends of S3 and S4 in D4, respectively.

Fig. 1 shows the whole-cell current traces recorded from the mutant and wild-type channels (Yang et al., 1994). The most striking change exhibited by all five PC mutants when compared with the wild type is a slowing of the current decay phase. Single-channel data indicate that this slowing is the result of a defect in the inactivation process (Fig. 3; see below). There is no difference in the activation phase of these currents between wild-type channel and mutant channels, and the current-voltage relationships are comparable in all channels.

The slowing of current inactivation can be expressed quantitatively as changes in the current inactivation time constant (τ_h) at different depolarization voltages (from −40 to 60 mV) (Fig. 2*A*). Although the inactivation process in whole-cell recordings from both the wild-type and all of the PC mutants could be fit by a single-exponential function at each membrane potential, the time constant for inactivation in the five mutant channels was shifted to slower values at all potentials. At −10 mV, for

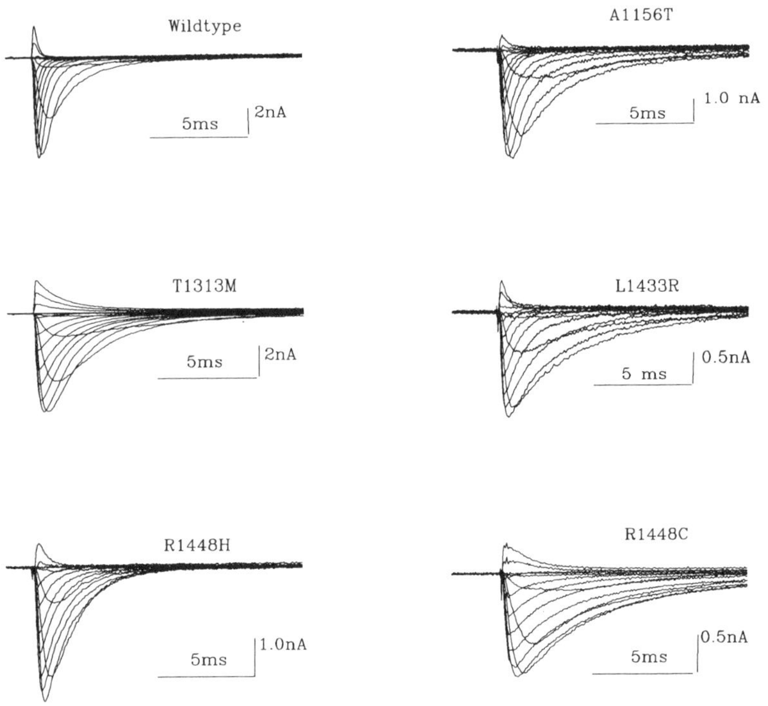

Figure 1. Whole-cell current traces recorded from wild-type and five different PC mutant channels expressed in tsA 201 cells. Currents were elicited by depolarization in steps of 10 mV from a holding potential of −90 mV. As compared with the wild-type channels, mutant channels show normal activation kinetics but inactivate more slowly.

example, the value of τ_h in the PC mutants ranged between two and five times slower than the wild type. In addition to the slowing of τ_h, several of these mutations also produced decreases in the voltage dependence of inactivation. This is especially obvious with the R1448C and R1448H mutations at voltages between −40 and 0 mV, a range over which the activation process takes place. Because the voltage dependence of inactivation is generally considered to derive from the voltage dependence of the preceding activation transitions (Aldrich, Corey, and Stevens, 1983; Cota and Armstrong, 1989), this suggests that there may be an uncoupling of inactivation from activation in these mutants (Chahine, George, Zhou, Ji, Sun, Barchi, and Horn, 1994). For the other PC mutants, τ_h is shifted to a proportionate extent at all voltages, retaining the approximate voltage dependence of the control channel. The lack of correlation between the degree of slowing in τ_h and extent of change in τ_h voltage dependence may indicate that conformational transitions in different parts of the channel structure can become rate limiting for the inactivation process under different conditions.

Although inactivation is slowed in these five PC mutant channels, recovery from inactivation is accelerated as compared with the wild-type channel (Fig. 2 *B*). These mutations decrease the voltage dependence of the recovery rate as well. This reduction is especially prominent in the R1448C, R1448H, and L1433R mutations.

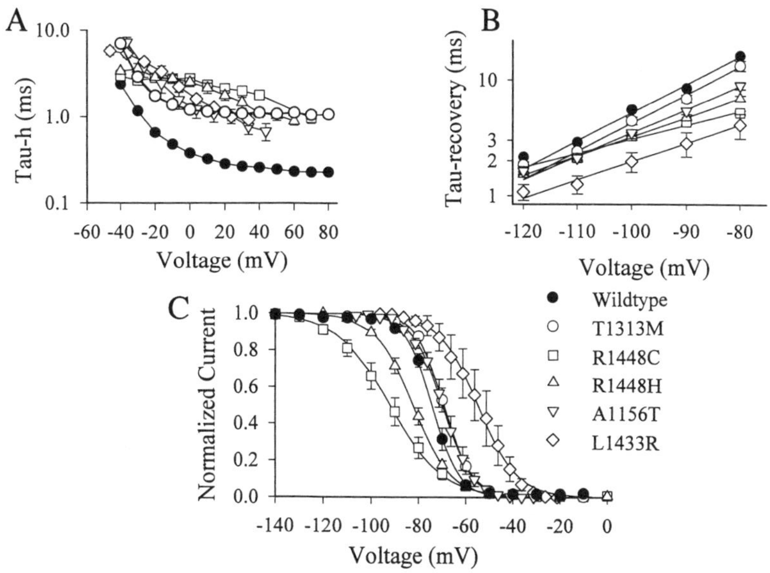

Figure 2. Inactivation time constants, recovery from inactivation and steady state inactivation curves from wild-type and PC mutant channels. (*A*) Inactivation time constants were estimated by fitting the inactivation phase of the sodium current to a single exponential: $I = A * \exp(-t/\tau) + A_\infty$. (*B*) Recovery was measured using a double pulse protocol: the first pulse was used to induce inactivation and, after various delays, a second pulse was used to assess the extent to which channels had recovered from inactivation. The solid curves are the best fits of recovery time constants at different holding potentials to the following equation: $\tau_r = \tau_o * \exp(k_r VF/RT)$, where $F/RT = 25$ mV. (*C*) Steady state inactivation was measured using a standard double pulse protocol. The solid curves are the best fits of the normalized current to a Boltzmann relationship: $I/I_{max} = 1/\{1 + \exp[z(V - V_{1/2})F/RT)$.

Steady state inactivation in these mutant channels is also significantly altered (Fig. 2 *C*). Both the slope and $V_{1/2}$ of the steady state inactivation curve (h_∞ curve) are affected. For the A1156T, T1313M, and L1433R mutations, the h_∞ curve is shifted ~15 mV toward more depolarized potentials. The R1448C and R1448H mutations, however, shift the curve in the hyperpolarized direction. Changes in the slope of the h_∞ curve are also variable: the slope is shallower in R1448C/H and L1433R but not significantly altered in A1156T and T1313M mutations, correlating with the effects of these mutations on the voltage dependence of recovery. Because the R1448C/H mutations and the mutations typified by T1313M share a common disease phenotype, kinetic rather than steady state factors must be of primary importance in determining the functional effects of these mutations in vivo.

The hallmark alteration in PC mutant channel gating, slowing of channel inactivation and increased rate of recovery from inactivation, is distinct from the appearance of a prominent slow gating mode in HyPP mutations (Cannon and Strittmatter, 1993; Cummins et al., 1993). This suggests that the A1156T mutation, identified in a patient with an ambiguous phenotype that shares clinical features of both HyPP and PC (McClatchey et al., 1992*a*), belongs to the category of PC. Given the variability of clinical features seen in families with periodic paralysis, the

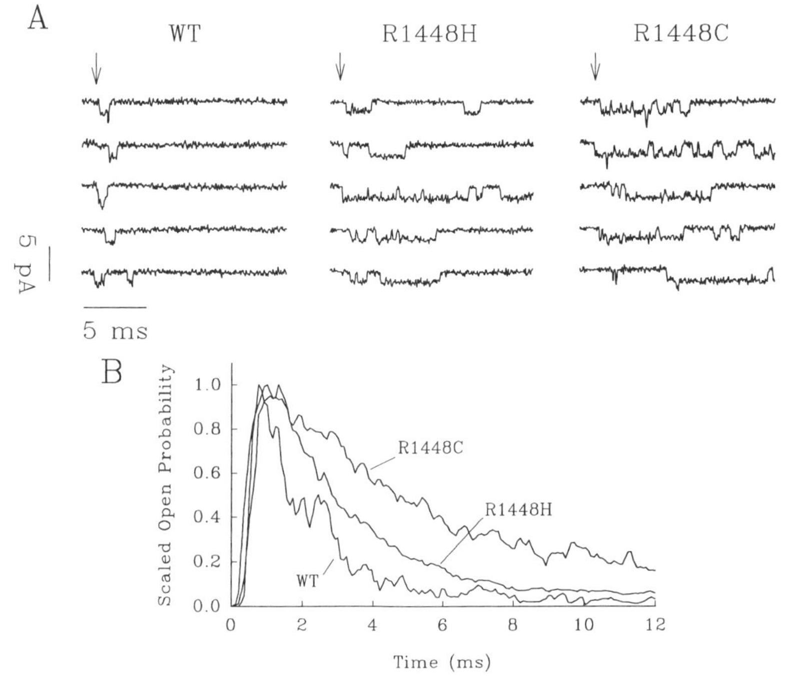

Figure 3. Single-channel recordings from wild-type and PC mutant channels. Recordings were done in the cell-attached configuration. Current was recorded at −20 mV from a holding potential of −80 mV. (*A*) Single-channel recordings from wild-type channel, and from R1448H and R1448C mutants. (*B*) Normalized opening probabilities for the three channels.

characteristics of channel gating may provide the most accurate basis for diagnostic classification of these diseases.

Single-Channel Studies

The slowing of the whole-cell current decay could be due to defects in either channel activation or inactivation. Although, as shown in Fig. 1, whole-cell current activation in mutant channels is not significantly altered, this point requires single-channel measurements for confirmation. Fig. 3 shows single-channel recordings from wild-type, R1448C, and R1448H mutant channels using the cell-attached patch configuration (Chahine et al., 1994). R1448C and R1448H mutant channels show little change in latency to first opening, but open repetitively during a single depolarizing pulse and exhibit a prolonged mean open time, indicating a defect in the channel inactivation process. Statistical analysis of multiple traces shows no evidence of temporal clustering that might indicate modal gating. Maximum likelihood analysis of the single channel data (Horn and Lange, 1983), based on the simplified kinetic scheme shown below,

$$\begin{array}{c} \qquad\qquad\quad I \\ \qquad\qquad \swarrow\!\!\nearrow \;\; \searrow\!\!\nwarrow \\ C_1 \rightleftharpoons C_2 \rightleftharpoons C_3 \rightleftharpoons O \end{array}$$

SCHEME I

indicates that the rate constants for transitions from the open to the inactivated state become much smaller while the rate constant for recovery from the inactivated state becomes larger in the mutant channels (Chahine et al., 1994). These changes are consistent with the changes in whole-cell currents described above, and suggest that fewer mutant channels are able to inactivate from the open state. Further, the more rapid rate of recovery from inactivation suggests that these mutations cause a destabilization of the inactivated state. The single-channel conductance of the mutant channels is not altered.

R1448 Mutations and External pH

Although R1448C and R1448H affect the same arginine residue, they differ considerably in the degree to which they alter channel gating. Because the positively charged Arg^{1448} is absolutely conserved in all sodium channels, these differences could reflect the relative impact of each substitution on this charge. At physiological pH (~7.4), cysteine is uncharged whereas histidine carries a partial positive charge. If charge neutralization plays a role in the action of these mutations, protonation of histidine by shifting extracellular pH would be expected to alter the magnitude of its effect on gating, and this is confirmed experimentally. When external pH is shifted to 7.8, a value at which histidine should carry little charge (the pK for histidine is between 6.1 and 6.8, depending on the local protein environment), the slowing of inactivation produced by R1448H is quantitatively similar to that seen with R1448C (Fig. 4*A*). In contrast, as histidine becomes protonated with decreasing pH, R1448H has progressively less effect on inactivation; at pH 6.2, the inactivation kinetics of the R1448H mutant channel are closer to those of the wild type. These results suggest that the positive charge carried by Arg^{1448} is important for normal gating of the channel. This charge may play a unique role in the coupling of the inactivation gate to the movement of the voltage sensor. However, alteration in charge may not be the sole factor involved because protonation of histidine does not totally reverse the slowing of channel inactivation. Steric factors may also play a subsidiary role in producing these effects.

Designed Mutations at 1433

Experiments with alteration of extracellular pH confirm the importance of the positive charge on Arg^{1448} for normal channel inactivation. Because the L1433R mutation should lie close to this residue near the extracellular surface of the protein in the tertiary structure, it is not unreasonable to postulate that the introduction of a positive charge at this previously neutral site is a major factor in its effect as well. To test this possibility, we constructed additional mutations at Leu^{1433} and compared their effects with L1433R.

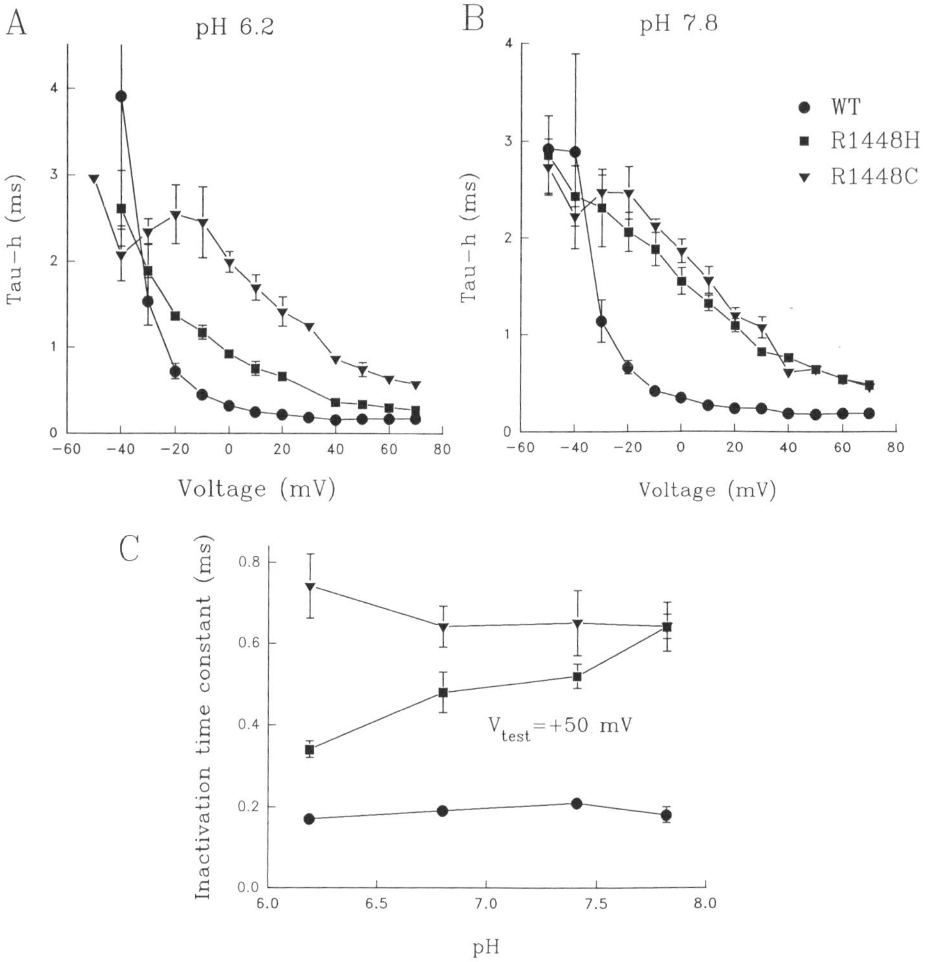

Figure 4. Effects of alterations of extracellular pH on the inactivation kinetics of Arg[1448] mutations. (*A*) Inactivation time constants at $pH_o = 6.2$. An acidic environment can cause protonation of histidine. (*B*) Inactivation time constants at $pH_o = 7.8$. At this pH, histidine should be little protonated. (*C*) τ_h at +50 mV as a function of extracellular pH. Changing pH within this range has little effect on the inactivation kinetics of either the wild-type or the R1448C mutant, but progressively alters the effects of the R1448H mutation from near control to levels comparable to R1448C.

Leucine and arginine differ in at least three properties: size of side chain, charge, and hydrophobicity (Greighton, 1993). Mutations were designed to examine each of these differences independently. They included L1433A, varying the size of the side chain without affecting polarity; L1433E and L1433K, probing the effects of charge; and L1433Q, introducing a neutral but polar side chain of intermediate size. Fig. 5 shows the effects of these mutations on the gating of the hSkM1 channel. Charge cannot be the sole factor responsible for the slowing of channel inactivation because the similarly charged lysine has less effect than arginine and the oppositely charged glutamic acid mutation affects the channel to a degree comparable to lysine. Change in the size of side chain may be an important factor because alanine, with the smallest side chain, has the least effect on inactivation, while the largest, arginine, has the greatest effect. However, the bulkier lysine affects channel inactivation less than smaller glutamine. Relative hydrophobicity might be the most important factor in determining the magnitude of the mutational effects because the observed increment in slowing with each mutant falls into the same order as does their relative hydrophobicity; $R > Q > K > E > A \approx L$ (Greighton, 1993). Because these mutations affect channel inactivation without significantly altering the voltage dependence of inactivation, S3 in D4 may participate in a channel inactivation transition downstream from the step that couples inactivation to the voltage-dependent transitions of activation.

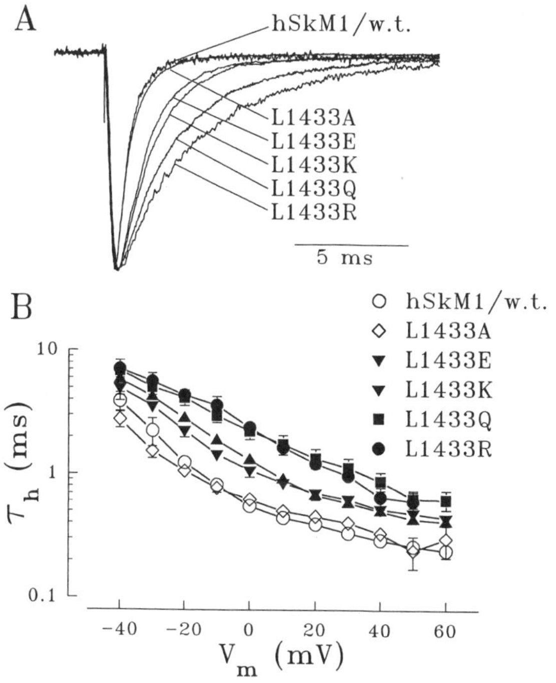

Figure 5. Normalized current traces and inactivation time constants in wild-type and Arg[1448] mutant channels. (*A*) Normalized current traces recorded at −10 mV from a holding potential of −90 mV. (*B*) Inactivation time constants (τ_h) at different depolarization voltages.

Analysis of the L1433R/R1448C Double Mutation

Since our analysis of the L1433R and R1448C mutations suggests that these mutations may produce their effects by different mechanisms, we explored the interaction between these mutations by constructing a double mutation containing both. Fig. 6 shows the effects of this double mutation on channel currents in transiently transfected tsA cells. The principal effect, again, is the slowing of channel inactivation. Interestingly, the effects of the double mutation resemble very closely those of R1448C alone and do not show additivity with the L1433R mutation. Besides the significant slowing in inactivation, the double mutation also causes a dramatic change in the voltage dependence of the inactivation rate that is indistinguishable from that seen with R1448C alone. These results suggest that for inactivation kinetics, the R1448C mutation has already produced a maximal effect on the rate of inactivation at a transition step that is rate limiting for the overall process. Because the dominant R1448C mutation alters the voltage dependence of τ_h, this

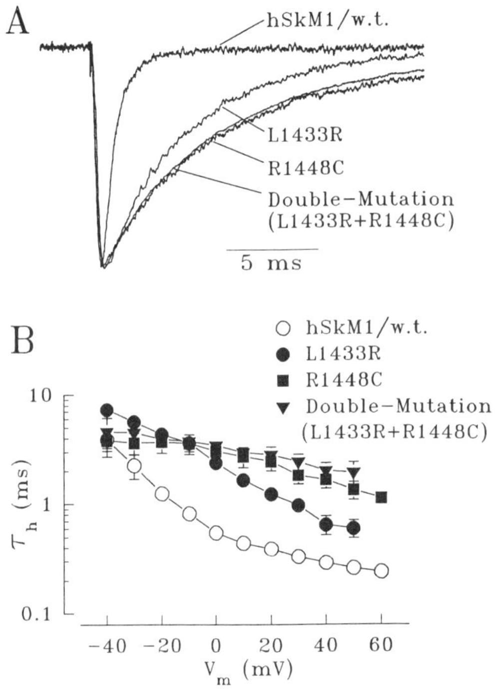

Figure 6. Normalized current traces and inactivation time constants in wild-type and double mutation (L1433R + R1448C) channels. (*A*) Normalized current traces recorded at −10 mV from a holding potential of −90 mV. (*B*) Inactivation time constants (T_h).

transition may involve coupling of inactivation to the movement of the activation domains during the activation-inactivation process.

In the steady state inactivation relationships, on the other hand, the double mutants behave in a manner that is indistinguishable from the L1433R mutation alone (Fig. 7). While the R1448C mutation shifts the h_∞ curve toward more hyperpolarizing potentials, the double mutant shifts this curve in the depolarizing direction to a point that superimposes on the h_∞ curve for L1433R alone. The transitions influenced by Leu[1433], while not rate limiting for the kinetics of inactivation when the channel is far from a steady state equilibrium, must exert a major influence on the steady state distribution of channels among different gating states. These effects of the double mutant on kinetics of channel inactivation and steady state inactivation suggest that S3 and S4 in D4 have different roles in the inactivation

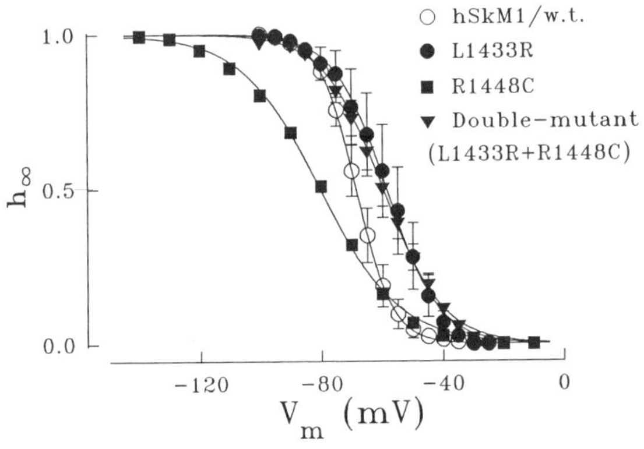

Figure 7. Steady state inactivation of sodium current in wild-type, L1433R, R1448C and double-mutation channels. Steady state inactivation was measured using a double-pulse protocol as in Fig. 2. The double-mutation resembles L1433R more closely than R1448C.

process, with the S4 being the primary initiator of this process. This conclusion is consistent with hypotheses proposed earlier (Stühmer, Conti, Suzuki, Wang, Noda, Yahagi, Kuba, and Numa, 1989).

Conclusions

Over the past few years, a growing list of mutations in the skeletal muscle voltage-dependent sodium channel have been identified that are implicated in the pathogenesis of diseases of excitability in human skeletal muscle (Table II). The molecular genetic analysis of these diseases, which include the periodic paralyses, paramyotonia congenita, and atypical myotonia, has led to a better understanding of their pathophysiology and a more rational approach to their diagnosis and treatment. However, the flow of information between the basic and the clinical sciences has been in both directions. Correlation of these mutations with their clinical phenotype and with the properties of individual channels in vitro has provided new insights into the basic elements of channel structure-function relationships, and has suggested new experiments to probe those relationships further.

Most of the mutations studied to date affect channel inactivation in one way or another. No mutations have been identified that affect only activation, and no mutations in the first repeat domain have surfaced. Undoubtedly, there are other groups of mutations associated with other muscle disease phenotypes which remain to be identified. More importantly, the recognition of these sodium channel mutations in muscle clearly points to the likely existence of a larger group of mutations involving voltage-dependent ion channels in the central nervous system. The heterogeneity of cell types and channel isoforms in the brain will make any predictions of clinical phenotype difficult, but the genetic epilepsies and various forms of mental retardation might make reasonable candidates for future study.

Acknowledgements

This work is in part supported by NIH grants NS-18103 (to R. L. Barchi) and AR-41691 (to R. Horn), and a grant from the Muscular Dystrophy Association (to R. L. Barchi). S. Ji is a Muscular Dystrophy Association postdoctoral research fellow. A. L. George is a Lucille P. Markey scholar.

References

Aldrich, R. W., D. P. Corey, and C. F. Stevens. 1983. A reinterpretation of mammalian sodium channel gating based on single channel recording. *Nature.* 306:436–441.

Barchi, R. L. 1988. Probing the molecular structure of the voltage-dependent sodium channel. *Annual Review of Neuroscience.* 11:455–495.

Barchi, R. L. 1993. Ion channels and disorders of excitation in skeletal muscle. *Current Opinion in Neurology and Neurosurgery.* 6:40–47.

Barchi, R. L. 1994. The muscle fiber and disorders of muscle excitability. *In* Basic Neurochemistry: Molecular, Cellular, and Medical Aspects. G. J. Siegel, B. Agranoff, R. W. Albers, and P. B. Molinoff, editors. Raven Press, Ltd., NY. 703–722.

Cannon, S. C., R. H. Brown, and D. P. Corey. 1991. A sodium channel defect in hyperkalemic periodic paralysis: Potassium-induced failure of inactivation. *Neuron.* 6:619–626.

Cannon, S. C., and S. M. Strittmatter. 1993. Functional expression of sodium channel mutations identified in families with periodic paralysis. *Neuron.* 10:317–326.

Chahine, M., A. L. George, Jr., M. Zhou, S. Ji, W. Sun, R. L. Barchi, and R. Horn. 1994. Sodium channel mutations in paramyotonia congenita uncouple inactivation from activation. *Neuron.* 12:281–294.

Cota, G., and C. M. Armstrong. 1989. Sodium channel gating in clonal pituitary cells: the inactivation step is not voltage dependent. *Journal of General Physiology.* 94:213–232.

Cummins, T. R., J. Zhou, F. J. Sigworth, C. Ukomadu, M. Stephan, L. J. Ptacek, and W. S. Agnew. 1993. Functional consequences of Na^+ channel causing hyperkalemic periodic paralysis. *Neuron.* 10:667–678.

Ebers, G. C., A. L. George, R. L. Barchi, S. S. Ting-Passador, R. G. Kallen, G. M. Lathrop, J. S. Beckmann, A. F. Hahn, W. F. Brown, R. D. Campbell, and A. J. Hudson. 1991. Paramyotonia congenita and hyperkalemic periodic paralysis are linked to the adult muscle sodium channel gene. *Annals of Neurology.* 30:810–816.

Fontaine, B., T. S. Khurana, E. P. Hoffman, G. A. P. Bruns, J. L. Haines, J. A. Trofatter, M. P. Hanson, J. Rich, H. McFarlane, D. M. Yasek, D. Romano, J. F. Guesella, and R. H. Brown. 1990. Hyperkalemic periodic paralysis and the adult muscle sodium channel α-subunit gene. *Science.* 250:1000–1002.

George, A. L. Jr., G. S. Iyer, R. Kleinfield, R. G. Kallen, and R. L. Barchi. 1993. Genomic organization of the human skeletal muscle sodium channel gene. *Genomics.* 15:598–606.

George, A. L., Jr., J. Komisarof, R. G. Kallen, and R. L. Barchi. 1991*a.* Primary structure of the adult human skeletal muscle voltage-dependent sodium channel. *Annals of Neurology.* 31:131–137.

George, A. L., Jr., D. H. Ledbetter, R. G. Kallen, and R. L. Barchi. 1991*b.* Assignment of a human skeletal muscle sodium channel α-subunit gene (SCN4A) to 17q23.1-25.3. *Genomics.* 9:555–556.

Greighton, T. E. 1993. Proteins: Structure and Molecular Properties. W. H. Freeman and Company, New York. 507 pp.

Heine, R., U. Pika, and F. Lehmann-Horn. 1993. A novel SCN4A mutation causing myotonia aggravated by cold and potassium. *Human Molecular Genetics.* 2:1349–1353.

Horn, R., and K. Lange. 1983. Estimating kinetic constants from single channel data. *Biophysical Journal.* 43:207–223.

Isom, L. L., K. S. De Jongh, D. E. Patton, R. F. X. Reber, J. Offord, H. Charbonneau, K. Walsh, A. L. Goldin, and W. A. Catterall. 1992. Primary structure and functional expression of the β_1 subunit of the rat brain sodium channel. *Science.* 256:839–842.

Jan, L. Y., and Y. N. Jan. 1989. Voltage-sensitive ion channels. *Cell.* 56:13–25.

Ji, S., W. Sun, A. L. George, Jr., R. Horn, and R. L. Barchi. 1994. Voltage-dependent regulation of modal gating in the rat SkM1 expressed in *Xenopus* oocytes. *Journal of General Physiology.* 104:625–643.

Kallen, R. G., Z.-H. Sheng, J. Yang, L. Chen, R. B. Rogart, and R. L. Barchi. 1990. Primary structure and expression of a sodium channel characteristic of denervated and immature rat skeletal muscle. *Neuron.* 4:233–242.

Koch, M. C., K. Ricker, M. Otto, T. Grimm, E. P. Hoffman, R. Rüdel, K. Bender, B. Zoll, P. S. Harper, and F. Lehmann-Horn. 1991. Confirmation of linkage of hyperkalemic periodic paralysis to chromosome 17. *Journal of Medical Genetics.* 28:583–586.

Koch, M. C., K. Steinmeyer, C. Lorenz, K. Ricker, F. Wolf, M. Otto, B. Zoll, F. Lehmann-Horn, K. Grzeschik, and T. J. Jentsch. 1992. The skeletal muscle chloride channel in dominant and recessive human myotonia. *Science.* 257:797–800.

Lehmann-Horn, F., R. Rüdel, and K. Ricker. 1993. Non-dystrophic myotonias and periodic paralysis. *Neuromuscular Disorders.* 3:161–168.

Lehmann-Horn, F., G. Küther, K. Ricker, P. Grafe, K. Ballanyi, and R. Rüdel. 1987*a*. Adynamia episodic hereditaria with myotonia: a non-inactivating sodium current and the effect of extracellular pH. *Muscle and Nerve.* 10:363–374.

Lehmann-Horn, F., R. Rüdel, K. Ricker. 1987*b*. Membrane defects in paramyotonia congenita (Eulenburg). *Muscle and Nerve.* 10:633–641.

Lehmann-Horn, F., R. Rüdel, K. Ricker, H. Lorkovic, R. Dengler, and H. C. Hopf. 1983. Two cases of adynamia episodica hereditaria: in vitro investigation of muscle cell membrane and contraction parameters. *Muscle and Nerve.* 6:113–121.

Lerche, H., R. Heine, U. Pika, A. L. George, Jr., N. Mitrovic, M. Browatzki, T. Weiss, M. Rivet-Bastide, C. Franke, M. Lomonaco, K. Ricker, and F. Lehmann-Horn. 1993. Human sodium channel myotonia: slowed channel inactivation due to substitutions for a glycine within the III-IV linker. *Journal of Physiology.* 470:13–22.

Makita, N., P. B. Bennett, Jr., and A. L. George, Jr. 1994. Voltage-gated Na^+ channel β_1 subunit mRNA expressed in adult human skeletal muscle, heart, and brain is encoded by a single gene. *Journal of Biological Chemistry.* 269:7571–7578.

McClatchey, A. I., D. McKenna-Yasek, D. Cros, H. G. Worthen, R. W. Kuncl, S. M. De Silva, D. R. Cornblath, J. F. Gusella, and R. H. Brown, Jr. 1992*a*. Novel mutations in families with unusual and variable disorders of the skeletal muscle sodium channel. *Nature Genetics.* 2:148–152.

McClatchey, A. I., P. Van den Bergh, M. A. Pericak-Vance, W. Raskind, C. Verellen, D. McKenna-Yasek, K. Rao, J. L. Haines, T. Bird, R. H. Brown, Jr., and J. F. Gusella, 1992*b*. Temperature-sensitive mutations in III–IV cytoplasmic loop region of the skeletal muscle sodium channel gene in paramyotonia congenita. *Cell.* 68:769–774.

Noda, M., T. Ikeda, T. Kayano, H. Suzuki, H. Takeshima, M. Kurasaki, H. Takahashi, and S. Numa. 1986. Existence of distinct sodium channel messenger RNAs in rat brain. *Nature.* 320:188–192.

Ptàček, L. J., A. L. George, Jr., R. L. Barchi, R. C. Griggs, J. E. Riggs, M. Robertson, and M. F. Leppert. 1992*a*. Mutations in an S4 segment of the adult skeletal muscle sodium channel cause paramyotonia congenita. *Neuron.* 8:891–897.

Ptàček, L. J., A. L. George, Jr., R. C. Griggs, R. Tawil, R. G. Kallen, R. L. Barchi, M. Robertson, and M. F. Leppert. 1991*a*. Identification of a mutation in the gene causing hyperkalemic periodic paralysis. *Cell.* 67:1021–1027.

Ptàček, L. J., L. Gouw, H. Kwiecinski, P. McManis, J. R. Mendell, R. J. Barohn, A. L. George, Jr., B. L. Barchi, M. Robertson, and M. F. Leppert. 1993. Sodium channel mutations in paramyotonia congenita and hyperkalemic periodic paralysis. *Annals of Neurology.* 33:300–307.

Ptàček, L. J., R. Tawil, R. C. Griggs, G. Meola, P. Mcmanis, R. J. Barohn, J. R. Mendell, C. Harris, R. Spitzer, F. Santiago, and M. F. Leppert. 1994. Sodium channel mutations in acetazolamide-responsive myotonia congenita, paramyotonia congenita, and hyperkalemic periodic paralysis. *Neurology.* 44:1500–1503.

Ptàček, L. J., R. Tawil, R. C. Griggs, D. Storvick, and M. Leppert. 1992*b*. Linkage of atypical myotonia congenita to a sodium channel locus. *Neurology.* 42:431–433.

Ptàček, L. J., J. S. Trimmer, W. S. Agnew, J. W. Roberts, J. H. Petajan, and M. Leppert. 1991*b*. Paramyotonia congenita and hyperkalemic periodic paralysis map to the same sodium channel gene locus. *American Journal of Human Genetics.* 49:851–854.

Ptàček, L. J., F. Tyler, J. S. Trimmer, W. S. Agnew, and M. Leppert. 1991*c*. Analysis in a large hyperkalemic periodic paralysis pedigree supports tight linkage to a sodium channel locus. *American Journal of Human Genetics.* 49:378–382.

Riggs, J. E. 1988. The periodic paralyses. *Neurologic Clinics.* 6:485–498.

Rojas, C. V., J. Wang, L. S. Schwartz, E. P. Hoffman, B. R. Powell, and R. H. Brown. 1991. A Met-to-Val mutation in the skeletal muscle Na^+ channel α-subunit in hyperkalemic periodic paralysis. *Nature.* 354:387–389.

Rüdel, R., and F. Lehmann-Horn. 1985. Membrane changes in cells from myotonia patients. *Physiological Reviews.* 65:310–356.

Rüdel, R., K. Ricker, and F. Lehmann-Horn. 1993. Genotype-phenotype correlations in human skeletal muscle sodium channel diseases. *Archives of Neurology.* 50:1241–1248.

Streib, E. W. 1991. Paramyotonia Congenita. *Seminars in Neurology.* 11:249–257.

Stühmer, W., F. Conti, H. Suzuki, X. D. Wang, M. Noda, N. Yahagi, H. Kubo, and S. Numa. 1989. Structural parts involved in activation and inactivation of the sodium channel. *Nature.* 339:597–603.

Trimmer, J. S., S. S. Cooperman, S. A. Tomiko, J. Y. Zhou, S. M. Crean, M. B. Boyle, R. G. Kallen, Z. Sheng, R. L. Barchi, F. J. Sigworth, R. H. Goodman, W. S. Agnew, and G. Mandel. 1989. Primary structure and functional expression of a mammalian skeletal muscle sodium channel. *Neuron.* 3:33–49.

Yang, N., S. Ji, M. Zhou, L. J. Ptàček, R. L. Barchi, R. Horn, and A. L. George, Jr. 1994. Sodium channel mutations in paramyotonia congenita exhibit similar biophysical phenotypes in vitro. *Proceedings of the National Academy of Sciences, USA.* 91:12785–12789.

Yang, J. S.-J., J. T. Sladky, R. G. Kallen, and R. L. Barchi. 1991. TTX-sensitive and TTX-insensitive sodium channel mRNA transcripts are independently regulated in adult skeletal muscle after denervation. *Neuron.* 7:421–427.

Zhou, J., J. F. Potts, J. S. Trimmer, W. S. Agnew, and F. J. Sigworth. 1991. Multiple gating modes and the effect of modulating factors on the μl sodium channel. *Neuron.* 7:775–785.

In vivo Sodium Channel Structure/Function Studies: Consecutive Arg1448 Changes to Cys, His, and Pro at the Extracellular Surface of IVS4

Jianzhou Wang,* Victor Dubowitz,‡ Frank Lehmann-Horn,§ Kenneth Ricker,§ Louis Ptacek,‖ and Eric P. Hoffman*

**Departments of Molecular Genetics and Biochemistry, Human Genetics, and Pediatrics University of Pittsburgh School of Medicine, Pittsburgh, Pennsylvania 15261; ‡Department of Paediatrics and Neonatal Medicine, Hammersmith Hospital, London, W12 ONN, United Kingdom; §Department of Applied Physiology, University of Ulm, D-89096 Ulm, Germany; and ‖Department of Neurology, University of Utah School of Medicine, Salt Lake City, Utah 84132*

Structure/function relationships in ion channels have been intensively studied through expression of cloned channel subunits in heterologous cellular environments. Considerable information has been gleaned via this approach. However, it is difficult to know if the residues and regions identified as important retain this prominent role in vivo: there are many differences between heterologous systems and functioning nerves and muscle in vivo, any one of which is likely to affect channel function. Examples of such variables include glycosylation status of the channel protein, association of muscle-specific membrane or cytoskeletal proteins, and fluctuations of intracellular and extracellular fluid milieu as a function of fluctuating cellular physiology. The identification of single amino acid changes in the voltage-sensitive muscle sodium channel α subunit in human and horse genetic disease has permitted a new approach to the study of structure/function relationships in ion channels. Importantly, the interactions between the environment and the abnormal channel can be studied in this in vivo system. Here we report the identification of a novel human sodium channel mutation (R1448P), which causes a severe type of cold-sensitive myotonia and weakness. This patient is compared to a series of other patients having R1448C, and R1448H mutations. We show that the severity of the amino acid change correlates with the severity of clinical symptoms. This data shows that different amino acid replacements in the extracellular surface of domain IV S4 are important for channel function, despite the paucity of heterologous expression data suggesting functional importance of this region. The extreme cold sensitivity of the proline subsitution at R1443 suggests that cold temperatures may affect the structural integrity of the channel, and that proline may destabilize the normal structure.

Introduction

A group of inherited neurological disorders share a propensity for involuntary repetitive firing of muscle (myotonia), with or without associated episodic weakness (periodic paralysis). Nondystrophic myotonias generally do not show progressive muscle destruction as a clinical feature. Nearly all of the inherited primary types of nondystrophic myotonia are transmitted within families as a dominant trait: patients are heterozygous, with both a normal and abnormal gene. Most dominantly inherited mutations cause a "change-of-function" of the corresponding protein product: the mutant gene can still produce a protein product, however the product does not function correctly. The abnormal protein initiates a cascade of events that leads to the clinical phenotype.

The nondystrophic myotonias have been divided into subgroups based on clinical and laboratory features (Rudel, 1986). Hyperkalemic periodic paralysis (HyperPP) shows attacks of weakness or paralysis provoked by rest after exercise or ingestion of potassium salt, with most patients showing evidence of interictal myotonia. First described in humans in the 1950's (Gamstorp, 1956), HyperPP is also prevalent in Quarter horses with ~1/200 (0.5%) of the 3 million registered horses having the trait (Spier, Carlson, Holliday, Cardinet, and Pickar, 1990). Paramyotonia congenita (PC) shows attacks of myotonia induced by low temperatures, associated with or followed by some weakness. Thomsen's myotonia shows myotonia most often accompanied by stiffness, without weakness or paralysis. Becker's myotonia is clinically similar to Thomsen's although it is more frequently associated with transient weakness. It is the only nondystrophic myotonia inherited as a recessive trait. Hypokalemic periodic paralysis does not show myotonia, shows reduced penetrance in women, and has attacks induced by carbohydrate or sodium intake, and insulin or epinephrine injection. Patients frequently show a progressive myopathy, and attacks decrease in severity and frequency with age.

Recently, the clinical subtypes of nondystrophic myotonias have resolved into three types of genetic disorders involving sodium, chloride, and calcium channels. Different change-of-function mutations of the voltage-sensitive sodium channel cause most cases of PC and HyperPP (both human and horse) (Rojas, Wang, Schwartz, Hoffman, Powell, and Brown, 1991; Ptacek, George, and Griggs, 1991; McClatchey, Van den Berg, Pericak-Vance, Raskind, Verellen, McKenna-Yasek, Rao, Haines, Bird, Brown, and Gusella, 1992; Rudolph, Spier, Byrn, Rojas, Bernoco, and Hoffman, 1992), loss-of-function mutations of the voltage-sensitive muscle chloride channel appear to cause many cases of Thomsen's and Becker's myotonia (Koch, Steinmeyer, Lorenz, Richer, Wolf, Otto, Zoll, Lehmann-Horn, Grzeschik, and Jentsch, 1992; George, Crackower, Abdalla, Hudson, and Ebers, 1993), and mutations of the α subunit of the dihydrophyridine (DHP) receptor have been found to cause hypokalemic periodic paralysis (Jurkat-Rott, Lehmann-Horn, Elbaz, Heine, Gregg, Hogan, Powers, Lapie, Vale-Santos, Weissenbach, and Fontaine, 1995; Ptacek, Tawil, Griggs, Engel, Layzer, Kwiecinski, McManis, Santiago, Moore, Fouad, Bradley, and Leppert, 1995).

Because of their crucial role in generation of action potentials in excitable tissues, the voltage-sensitive sodium channels have held the rapt attention of biologists for decades. Mapping the regions involved in channel activation, inactivation, and ion selection has been an intense area of channel research, yet much remains poorly understood. To date, research on these processes has been largely acquired through the formulation of theoretical models, with subsequent experimental testing of these models. A particularly informative recent experimental strategy has been the theoretical deduction of the structure of voltage-sensitive channels based upon their primary sequences, and the experimental functional testing of channel proteins containing amino acid substitutions by in vitro expression and electrophysiological recording.

An alternative approach is to empirically identify organisms with functional deficiencies of motor response or movement, and identify the corresponding gene and protein. The advantage of this approach is that the effect of protein dysfunction is seen in vivo. Recent advances in studying molecular basis of inherited myotonic disorders have facilitated the use of human and animal disease as tools for the understanding of basic biological processes, such as structure/function relationships. Through this work, we have shown that the identification and characterization of genes disrupting motor response or movement directly address relevant human diseases, and also address questions of basic biology.

Here we compare a series of patients with consecutive amino acid replacements of arginine in the extracellular surface of domain IV, transmembrane segment 4. The extreme temperature sensitivity of a proline substitution in this position suggests that this region is important for the structural integrity of the channel, and that cold temperatures may alter the stability of the normal structure.

Methods

Genomic DNA was isolated from peripheral blood leukocytes (Higuchi, 1989), and each of the 24 exons of the adult skeletal muscle sodium channel α subunit (SCN4) gene were scanned for possible mutations using PCR-SSCP as previously described (Baquero, Ayala, Wang, Curless, Feero, Hoffman, and Ebeid, 1995). PCR products showing aberrant conformers were cloned into M13 vector and sequenced from both directions (Rojas et al., 1991). Ligase chain reaction (LCR) was performed as previously described (Feero, Wang, Barany, Zhou, Todorovic, Conwit, Galloway, Hausmanowa-Petrusewicz, Fidzianska, Aratiata, Wessel, Sillen, Marks, Hartlage, and Hoffman, 1993).

Patients

R1448P: One Patient Was Studied

Patient VD1. This eight-year-old girl has been with a foster mother since the age of 3. It was already noted at that time that she had a tendency to walk on her toes and had marked difficulty with walking in the cold, which also produced spasm on closure of her eyelids with delayed opening, particularly when exposed to cold. She was so cold sensitive that even a tepid bath could produced marked muscle spasm. There was at times also slurring of her speech. Cold also induced at times a feeling of being floppy or weak but this was difficult to quantify in terms of severity or duration and there were no overt attacks of paralysis. She also experienced some stiffness on walking in the morning.

On clinical assessment here was no demonstrable voluntary myotonia of the hands, but delayed opening of the eyes after tight closure (lid lag), and marked percussion myotonia of the tongue after a finger tap. Her muscle power was good and she was able to rise from the floor without difficulty. There were a few spontaneous myotonic discharges on electromyography. A diagnosis of paramyotonia congenita was made, with the possibility of an associated mild periodic paralysis.

She has a brother who is clinically normal and two sisters, possibly by a different father, who are said to be normal. There is little information on the biological parents, but the father may have had a Raynaud's phenomenon of the hands in the cold.

R1448H: Three Patients from Two Unrelated Families Were Studied

Family K1800. Published clinical data (Riggs, Griggs, and Moxley, 1977) was available for an affected 25-year-old male who was subsequently found to have the R1448H mutation. This patient reported nocturnal attacks of weakness which were noted in the early morning since he was 12. The weakness improved with activity. A 5- to 10-min exposure to cold induced marked myotonia, with subsequent dramatic decrease in strength over the next 20 min. Attacks were not induced by rest after exercise. Challenge with potassium ingestion (9 g) caused an strong increase in eye lid myotonia and slight increase in grip myotonia, but no episode of weakness. The patient showed hypertrophied calves and fasciculations (spontaneous myotonia) of muscles. Administration of acetazolamide (250 mg every 6 h for 2 d) abolished myotonia, but increased weakness.

Family PC18. This 36-year-old male and his son (three-years old) reported that opening of the eyelids is difficult, in particular after a strong closure (e.g., when sneezing) or repeated closures. Worsening of myotonia with continued exercise (i.e., paradoxical myotonia) was also present in other muscles after cooling. On intensive exercise and cooling, the stiffness was followed by weakness. Spontaneous attacks of weakness were not reported. On examination, the patient showed hypertrophy of the proximal muscles. Myotonia was present in eyelids, tongue, and limb muscles, but percussion myotonia only in the thumb. Electromyography revealed myotonic activity.

R1448C: Three Patients from Three Unrelated Families Were Studied

Family PC2. Published clinical data was available for seven out of nine family members carrying the mutation (=family D [Ricker, Haass, Rudel, B'hlen, and Mertens, 1980; Ricker, B'hlen, and Rohkamm, 1983]). All showed myotonia in the second decade that was present at all times, though rarely incapacitating. The myotonia was most evident after rest, and would improve with activity. The myotonia was greatly exacerbated by even minor cooling of the muscle, with flaccid paralysis after. Two patients noted exacerbation of myotonia by pregnancy. Cold-induced myotonia was present at a younger age than the symptomatic myotonia in a warm-environment. All affected family members reported spontaneous attacks of generalized weakness which was most pronounced in the legs, and would last from hours to days. When measured serum potassium was increased during these attacks which often occurred in the morning (i.e., hyperkalemic periodic paralysis). Ingestion of potassium (120 mmol KCl by mouth) did induce such attacks of weakness. Tocainide was effective in both reducing myotonia and preventing cold-induced weakness whereas acetazolamide prevented episodes of hyperkalemic weakness (Ricker et al., 1980). Serum creatine kinase was slightly above the upper limit of normal range in all affected family members.

Family PC33. This 51-year-old male and his son (27-years old) reported cold-induced stiffness of face and hands, e.g., stiff tongue when eating ice cream. Occasionally, the stiffness gave way to weakness and the cooled muscles may remain paralyzed for several hours after rewarming. Both experienced spontaneous attacks of weakness, especially of the legs during rest after exercise. All other affected family members were reported to have the same combination of cold-induced symptoms and spontaneous attacks of weakness. Physical examination showed normal muscle relaxation and no percussion myotonia at warm environment but stiffness of muscles after cooling. The index patient revealed slight muscle atrophy and paresis in the shoulder girdle and in the lower legs.

Family K1637. This 49-year old female reported episodes of weakness beginning ~8 yr of age, and sensitivity to cold temperatures beginning before age 5 yr. Episodes of weakness were experienced after rest, usually during the day after sitting, and lasted 1–4 h, and were often accompanied by pain. Activity could ward off attacks. The patient complained of urgent urination during attacks. She complains that her "tongue gets big" when ingesting cold drinks or food, and myotonia of the hands in cold water lasting 30–40 min. The patient reported that carbohydrate intake seemed to ablate attacks. Pregnancy did not exacerbate attacks, and in fact may have ablated them. Muscle biopsy showed formation of intracellular vacuoles after cooling of the muscle before biopsy. The patient reported that emotional stress, hunger, and exercise all seemed to promote attacks of weakness more often than low temperatures.

Family K2125. This 44-year old male reported that his parents noted eyelid myotonia from infancy, and subsequently showed myotonic contractures of eyelids, mouth, hands, and feet upon exposure to cold temperatures. He tells an amusing story of his family members at family reunions eating ice cream and "locking up their entire faces." He reports that episodes of weakness are more debilitating than the cold-induced myotonia, which often occurred in the morning. His most severe attack was during a cold bath after strenous sports activity, where he fell asleep only to awaken with labored breathing and complete limb paralysis. He was able to feebly call for help, and was rescued from sinking into the water by his brother. The frequency of attacks of weakness increased with age, with two attacks per month with weakness persisting for 3–4 d.

Results

Identification of Arg1448Pro Mutation

The patient with severe cold induced general weakness (VD1) was tested for two common mutations of the sodium channel gene by LCR (Feero et al., 1993). This patient did not have these previously identified HyperPP sodium channel mutations. To detect possible unknown sodium channel mutations, we scanned the entire sodium channel gene (24 exons) with PCR-SSCP analysis. A unique conformer in exon 24 of this patient's sodium channel gene was detected (Fig. 1 *A*). The PCR product, which corresponds to amino acid 1429–1518, was then cloned into M13 vector, and 10 clones of this patient's PCR product were sequenced. Sequence analysis showed a C to G substitution in 4 of 10 clones (Fig. 1 *B*), which resulted in an arginine to a proline change at amino acid position 1448 (Wang, Rojas, Zhou, Schwartz, Nicholas, and Hoffman, 1992). This Arg1448Pro change is at exactly the same amino acid position, at which two previously identified PC mutations (Arg1448His and Arg1448Cys) were located (Fig. 2). According to current structure models of the sodium channels, Arg1448 is localized in domain IV, near the extracellular surface of transmembrane segment S4.

Comparison of Clinical Presentation of Patients with Three Different Mutations at Same Amino Acid Position in Adult Skeletal Muscle Sodium Channel

The identification of a patient with a novel arginine to proline change (patient VD1) permitted the comparison of a series of paramyotonia patients with different single amino acid changes at position 1448 in the extracellular surface of the sodium channel. Detailed clinical records were obtained for two unrelated patients with an arginine to histidine change (families K1800, PC18), and four unrelated patients with an arginine to cysteine change (families PC2, PC33, K1637, and K2125) (Table I). There were similarities between patients with all three mutations: all showed an age of onset which was variable but invariably within the first decade, all showed cold-induced stiffness, and all showed percussion myotonia.

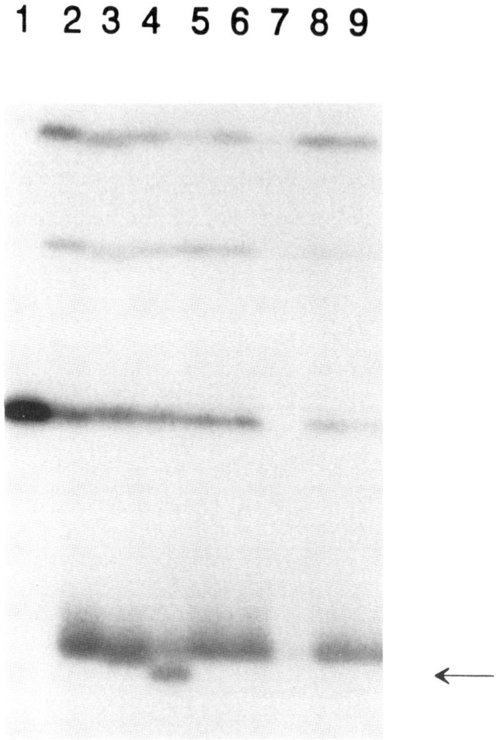

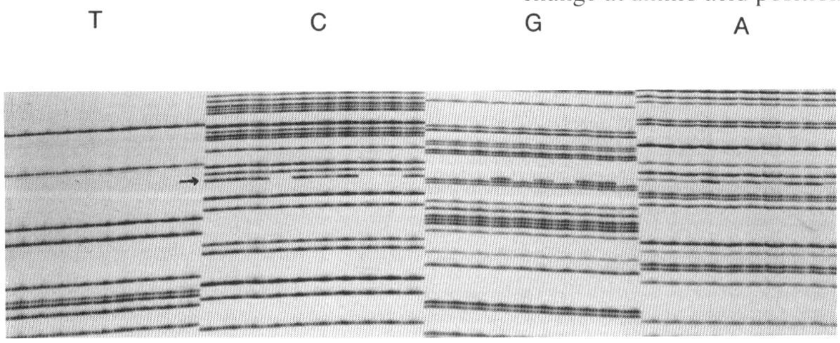

Figure 1. Molecular analysis of paramyotonia patient VD1, a patient extremely sensitive to cold temperatures. (*A*) Shown is SSCP analysis of sodium channel sequence corresponding to part of exon 24 (amino acids 1429–1518) from myotonia patients (lanes *3–9*). Six of seven patients showed the normal patterns of conformers (lanes *3, 5–9*), whereas patient VD1 (lane *4*) showed a unique pattern of SSCP conformers (*arrow*). Double-stranded and single-stranded PCR products from a normal individual are also shown as controls (lanes *1* and *2*).

(*B*) Shown is sequence analysis of the exon 24 SSCP conformers shown in *A*. The PCR product showing the unique conformers for exon 24 by SSCP was cloned into M13 vector and 10 clones were sequenced. A C to G substitution was found in 4 of 10 clones. This C to G substitution resulted in an arginine to a proline change at amino acid position 1448.

TABLE I
Clinical Presentation and Molecular Genetic Data for Patients from Seven Pedigrees

Mutation	Pedigree	Presenting symptoms	Myotonia			Attacks of weakness and/or paralysis			Current age	Interictal symptoms
			Spontaneous	Cold	Percussion	Frequency	Duration	Induced by		
R1448P	PC VD1	Severe cold-induced stiffness followed by weakness	++	++++	++	<1/mo	Hours	Low temperature	8	Fixed deformity of ankles and toe walking
R1448H	K1800	Cold-induced stiffness followed by weakness	no	++	+	Severe: 1/yr Mild: 1/mo	Days–weeks	Rest after exercise, alcohol	25	No
R1448H	PC18	Exercise and cold-induced stiffness followed by weakness	no	++	+	No	No	No	36	Proximal muscle hypertrophy
R1448C	PC2	Muscle stiffness at rest, and greatly exacerabted by cold	++	+++	+	<1/mo	Hours–days	Low temperature, potassium	40	No
R1448C	PC33	Cold-induced stiffness of face and hand	+	++	+	<1/mo	Hours	Rest after exercise, low temperature	51	Slight muscle atrophy and weakness in the shoulder girdle and lower legs
R1448C	K1637	Cold-induced weakness	+	++	+	<1/mo	1–4 h	Exercise, emotional stress hunger, and less frequently cold	49	No
R1448C	K2125	Cold-induced stiffness, exercise, and cold-induced general weakness	+	++	+	2/mo (increased with age)	3–4 d	Exercise and low temperature	44	No

The major difference between the three mutations was the increased clinical severity of the proline substitution compared to the histidine and cystein mutations. The proline substitution is the most dramatic amino acid substition, both resulting in the loss of a positive charge near the proposed ion conducting pore (S4 segment), and probably causing structural changes in the channel (proline is most often associated with bends in the polypeptide chain). Consistent with the severity of the amino acid change, the patient's clinical phenotype was the most severe of the seven patients studied in detail. This young girl showed extreme sensitivity to cold, with even tepid water causing marked muscle spasms (spontaneous myotonia). She also showed fixed deformity of her ankles with toe walking, suggesting marked myotonia and/or fixed weakness from a young age. Her percussion myotonia was also more dramatic than patients with the other amino acid changes.

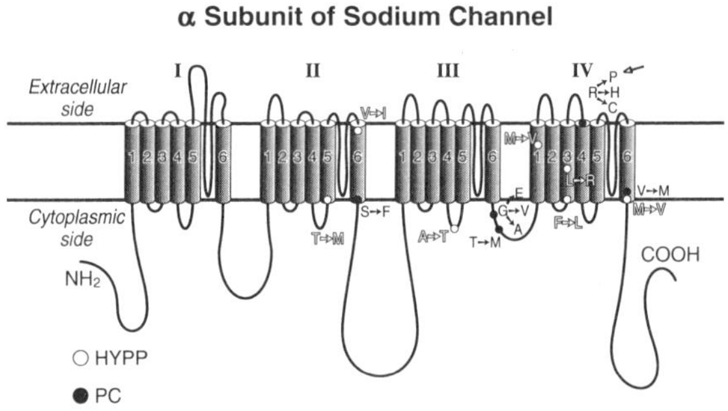

Figure 2. Summary of sodium channel mutations identified to date. Shown are the single amino acid changes of the adult skeletal muscle sodium channel protein that have been identified in hyperkalemic periodic paralysis (HYPP) and paramyotonia congenita (PC) patients. The hollow arrow at the top of the diagram indicates the position of the arginine to proline mutation described in this report (R1448P), with the two additional amino acid changes found in other patients (R1448C, R1448H). The clinical features of the patients with different mutations at R1448 are compared and contrasted in this report.

Note that some of the mutations shown do not cause "pure" HYPP or PC, and patients with these mutations instead show overlap symptoms or simple myotonia.

Discussion

Structure/Function Correlations in the Voltage-sensitive Ion Channelopathies: In vitro Mutagenesis Studies Vs In vivo Patient Studies

With advances in molecular biology and patch clamp recording techniques, in vitro expression analysis has become the method of choice for the study of structure/function relationships in voltage-dependent ion channels. Site directed mutagenesis has been extensively used to produce specific changes in channel primary structure, with the mutant channels then introduced into *Xenopus* oocytes or mammalian cell lines via expression vectors.

Although these in vitro studies have achieved considerable success, they have several limitations. First, these studies are usually directed by hypothetical structural models and may miss functionally important regions not suggested by the models. Second, the expression systems used are oocytes or transformed cell lines: these experimental systems undoubtedly have dramatically different intracellular and membrane environments as compared to the sodium channel's natural host, myofibers or neurons. The differences include presence of the different subunits, membrane structure, tissue-specific posttranslation modifications, among others. Our studies of the molecular basis of ion channelopathies in humans and horses have provided an important complementary approach to channel structure and function by studying channel dysfunction in vivo.

Voltage-dependent activation and inactivation are the key functional features of the voltage-dependent sodium channels. Voltage-dependent activation controls the opening of the sodium channel in response to initial depolarization. Inactivation shifts the channel from an open, ion-conducting state to a closed, inactivated state during a sustained depolarization. Mapping the regions involved in activation and inactivation has been one of major focuses of in vitro structure/function studies.

One model of sodium channel inactivation recently supported by extensive data from in vitro structure/function studies (Catterall, 1992) proposes that voltage-dependent activation or opening of the channel occurs because of movement of positively charged S4 segments within the membrane. Thus, selected amino acid substitutions in the S4 segments either shift the voltage dependence of Na channel activation, or alter its steepness; for this reason, these positively charged S4 helices have been considered to be voltage sensors. In this model, rapid or fast inactivation is attributed to movement of the III-IV cytoplasmic loop into the pore (West, Patton, Scheuer, Wang, Goldin, and Catterall, 1992). This "inactivation gate" is believed to interact with docking sites within the cytoplasmic end of the channel pore. Antibodies against this region and single amino acid substitutions within this region can abolish inactivation or slow its rate (Vassilev, Scheuer, and Catterall, 1988, 1989; Stuhmer, Conti, Suzuki, Wang, Noda, Yahagi, Kubor, and Numa, 1989; Moorman, Kirsch, Brown, and Joho, 1990). The location and identity of the putative docking sites have not been identified. Data from studies of both K^+ and Na^+ channel suggests there may also be a slow component of inactivation which, by contrast with fast inactivation, is not mediated by the III-IV loop (Hoshi, Zagotta, and Aldrich, 1991; Choi, Aldrich, and Yellen, 1991; Zagotta, Hoshi, and Aldrich, 1990). Rather, slow inactivation probably depends primarily on changes in the conformation of regions of the channel at the extracellular face of the membrane.

Do the mutations detected in myotonia and periodic paralysis patients occur in amino acids previously defined as functionally important by biophysical studies? The few mutations causing hyperkalemic periodic paralysis tend to arise in amino acid residues located within the membrane; one exception is a residue near the extracellular face of S4. It is less easy to understand how these affect inactivation. One possibility is that those located near the cytoplasmic surface affect potential docking sites for the inactivation gate, destabilizing or inhibiting inactivation: consistent with this hypothesis is the location of three hyperkalemic periodic paralysis mutations at the intracellular face of the plasma membrane. The location of the three III-IV loop mutations causing myotonia of varying severities correlates well with the purported function of this region as an "inactivation gate." Indeed, the mutations disrupt a -gly-gly- pair proposed to be a hinge for pivoting of the loop.

The amino acid changes causing paramyotonia congenita are diversely situated in the channel. Some are located in either the III-IV cytoplasmic loop or superficially at the extracellular end of S4, including the novel arginine to proline substitution identified in this report (R1448H,C,P) (Fig. 2). While the effect of the III-IV cytoplasmic may be easily explained as an impaired inactivation gate, the functional significance of the S4 mutations, one of which is a novel nonconservative change described in this report (R1448P) is less clear. Recent electrophysiological studies on

R1448H/C sodium channels expressed in a mammalian cell line, performed with patch clamp methods, revealed that this arginine residue is important for fast inactivation (Catine, George, Zhou, Ji, Sun, Barchi, and Horn, 1994). The authors reported altered channel kinetics and proposed a model in which inactivation is uncoupled from activation. Under the experimental conditions of voltage clamped membrane patches, low temperature had no direct effect on the expressed mutant sodium channels. The novel proline mutation identified here has not yet been studied by patch clamping. Proline is known to have a dramatic influence on the secondary structure of polypeptides. Also, the normal amino acid in this position has a positive charge (arginine) whereas proline carries no charge. Thus, the R1448P changes the charge of this highly conserved region, in addition to having a potentially dramatic effect on the secondary/tertiary structure of the channel. The remarkable sensitivity of this abnormal channel to temperature is more easily rationalized by structural effects of the proline rather than charge effects.

Many other questions remain concerning the functional effects of these mutations. Perhaps most challenging is an explanation of why extracellular K^+ ions can induce the failure of inactivation thought to underly the pathogenesis of either myotonia or inexcitability and paralysis. In any case, it remains very likely that the analysis of mutations causing these diseases has identified critical regions of the Na^+ channel not previously thought to be functionally important for channel activation or inactivation.

References

Baquero J. L., R. A. Ayala, J. Wang, R. G. Curless, G. W. Feero, E. P. Hoffman, and G. Ebeid. 1995. Hyperkalemic periodic paralysis with cardiac dysrhythmia: a novel sodium channel mutation? *Annals of Neurology*. In press.

Catterall, W. A. 1992. Cellular and molecular biology of channels. *Physiological Reviews.* 72:S15–S48.

Chahine, M., A. L. George, M. Zhou, S. Ji, W. Sun, R. L. Barchi, and R. Horn. 1994. Sodium channel mutations in paramyotonia congenita uncouple inactivation from activation. *Neuron.* 12:281–294.

Choi, K. L., R. W. Aldrich, and G. Yellen. 1991. Tetraethylammonium blockage distinguishes two inactivation mechanisms in voltage-activated K^+ channels. *Proceedings of the National Academy of Sciences, USA.* 88:5092–5095.

Feero, W. G., J. Wang, F. Barany, J. Zhou, S. M. Todorovic, R. Conwit, G. Galloway, I. Hausmanowa-Petrusewicz, A. Fidzianska, K. Arahata, H. B. Wessel, A. Sillen, H. G. Marks, P. Hartlage, H. Hayakawa, and E. P. Hoffman. 1993. Hyperkalemic periodic paralysis: rapid molecular diagnosis and relationship of genotype to phenotype in 12 families. *Neurology.* 43:668–673.

Gamstorp, I. 1956. Adynamia episodica hereditaria. *Acta Paediatrica Scandinavica.* 108(Suppl.): 1–126.

George, A. L., M. A. Crackower, J. A. Abdalla, A. J. Hudson, and G. C. Ebers. 1993. Molecular basis of Thomsen's disease (autosomal dominant myotonia congenita). *Nature Genetics.* 3:305–310.

Higuchi, R. 1989. Rapid, efficient DNA extraction for PCR from cells or blood. *In* Amplifications: A Forum for PCR Users. Cetus Corporation 1–3.

Hoshi, T., W. M. Zagotta, and R. W. Aldrich. 1991. Two types of inactivation in *Shaker* K^+ channels: effects of alternations in the carboxy-terminal region. *Neuron.* 7:547–556.

Jurkat-Rott, K., F. Lehmann-Horn, A. Elbaz, R. Heine, R. G. Gregg, K. Hogan, P. A. Powers, P. Lapie, J. E. Vale-Santos, J. Weissenbach, and B. Fontaine. 1995. A calcium chanel mutation causing hypokalemic periodic paralysis. *Human Molecular Genetics.* In press.

Koch, M. C., K. Steinmeyer, C. Lorenz, K. Ricker, F. Wolf, M. Otto, B. Zoll, F. Lehmann-Horn, K. Grzeschik, and T. J. Jentsch. 1992. The skeletal muscle chloride channel in dominant and recessive human myotonia. *Science.* 257:797–800.

McClatchey A. I., P. Van den Bergh, M. A. Pericak-Vance, W. Raskind, C. Verellen, D. McKenna-Yasek, K. Rao, J. L. Haines, T. Bird, R. H. Brown, and J. F. Gusella. 1992. Temperature-sensitive mutations in the III-IV cytoplasmic loop region of the skeletal muscle sodium channel gene in paramyotonia congenita. *Cell.* 68:769–774.

Moorman, J. R., G. E. Kirsch, A. M. Brown, and R. H. Joho. 1990. Changes in sodium channel gating produced by point mutations in a cytoplasmic linker. *Science.* 250:688–691.

Ptacek, L. J., A. L. George, and R. C. Griggs. 1991. Identification of a mutation in the gene causing hyperkalemic periodic paralysis. *Cell.* 67:1021–1027.

Ptacek, L. J., R. Tawil, R. C. Griggs, A. G. Engel, R. B. Layzer, H. Kwiecinski, P. G. McManis, L. Santiago, M. Moore, G. Fouad, P. Bradley, and M. F. Leppert. 1995. Dihydropyridine receptor mutations cause hypokalemic periodic paralysis. *Cell.* In press.

Ricker, K., A. Haass, R. Rudel, R. B'hlen, and H. G. Mertens. 1980. Successful treatment of paramyotonia congenita (Eulenburg). Muscle stiffness and weakness prevented by tocainide. *Journal of Neurology, Neurosurgery and Psychiatry.* 43:268–271.

Ricker, K., R. B'hlen, and R. Rohkamm. 1983. Different effectiveness of tocainide and hydrochlorothiazide in paramyotonia congenita with hyperkalemic episodic paralysis. *Neurology.* 33:1615–1618.

Riggs, J. E., R. C. Griggs, and R. T. Moxley. 1977. Acetazolamide-induced weakness in paramyotonia congenita. *Annals of Internal Medicine.* 86:169–174.

Rojas, C. V., J. Wang, L. S. Schwartz, E. P. Hoffman, B. R. Powell, and R. H. Brown. 1991. A methionine to valine mutation in the skeletal muscle sodium channel alpha-subunit in human hyperkalemic periodic paralysis. *Nature.* 354:387–389.

Rudel, R. 1986. The pathophysiologic basis of the myotonias and the periodic paralyses. *In* Myology: Basic and Clinical. A. G. Engel and B. Q. Banker, editors. McGraw-Hill, New York. 1297–1311.

Rudolph, J. A., S. J. Spier, G. Byrn, C. V. Rojas, D. Bernoco, and E. P. Hoffman. 1992. Periodic paralysis in Quarter Horses: a sodium channel mutation disseminated by selective breeding. *Nature Genetics.* 2:144–147.

Spier, S. J., G. P. Carlson, T. A. Holliday, G. H. Cardinet, and J. G. Pickar. 1990. Hyperkalemic periodic paralysis in horses. *Journal of American Veterinary Medicine Association.* 197:1009–1017.

Stuhmer, W., F. Conti, H. Suzuki, X. Wang, M. Noda, N. Yahagi, H. Kubo, and S. Numa. 1989. Structural parts involved in activation and inactivation of the sodium channel. *Nature.* 339:597–603.

Vassilev, P. M., T. Scheuer, and W. A. Catterall. 1988. Identification of an intracellular peptide segment involved in sodium channel inactivation. *Science.* 241:1658–1661.

Vassilev, P. M., T. Scheuer, and W. A. Catterall. 1989. Inhibition of inactivation of single sodium channels by a site-directed antibody. *Proceedings of the National Academy of Sciences, USA.* 86:8147–8151.

Wang, J., C. V. Rojas, J. Zhou, L. S. Schwartz, N. Nicholas, and E. P. Hoffman. 1992. Sequence and genomic structure of the human adult skeletal muscle sodium channel alpha subunit gene on 17q. *Biochemical and Biophysical Research Communications.* 182:794–801.

West, J. W., D. E. Patton, T. Scheuer, Y. Wang, A. L. Goldin, and W. A. Catterall. 1992. A cluster of hydrophobic amino acid residues required for fast Na^+ channel inactivation. *Proceedings of the National Academy of Sciences, USA.* 89:10910–10914.

Zagotta, W. N., T. Hoshi, and R. W. Aldrich. 1990. Restoration of inactivation in mutants of *Shaker* potassium channels by peptide derived from ShB. *Science.* 250:568–571.

Chapter 4

Disorders of Calcium Channels

The Role of the Skeletal Muscle Ryanodine Receptor (RYR1) Gene in Malignant Hyperthermia and Central Core Disease

David H. MacLennan and Michael S. Phillips

Banting and Best Department of Medical Research, University of Toronto, Charles H. Best Institute, Toronto, Ontario, Canada M5G1L6

The Ca^{2+} Release Channel of Skeletal Muscle Sarcoplasmic Reticulum

The sarcoplasmic reticulum is the major regulator of Ca^{2+} concentrations in skeletal muscle (Carafoli, 1987). Ca^{2+} is pumped into the sarcoplasmic reticulum by a Ca^{2+} transport ATPase to initiate relaxation, stored in the junctional terminal cisternae in association with calsequestrin, and released through a Ca^{2+} release channel to bind to troponin in the thin filament, initiating muscle contraction. Ca^{2+} also binds to phosphorylase kinase, activating glycolytic pathways and the resynthesis of ATP to replenish that used during contraction.

The Ca^{2+} release channel of the sarcoplasmic reticulum is a tetrameric protein complex constructed from four identical 565-kD subunits (Wagenknecht, Grassucci, Frank, Saito, Inui, and Fleischer, 1989). Single-channel measurements in planar bilayers have shown that Ca^{2+} release is mediated by a ligand-gated channel with a conductance >100 pS in 50 mM Ca^{2+} (Smith, Coronado, and Meissner, 1985). Transmembrane sequences are located in the COOH-terminal fifth of each subunit and the remainder of the subunit is probably cytoplasmic, bridging the gap between the sarcoplasmic reticulum and the transverse tubule (Takeshima, Nishimura, Matsumoto, Ishida, Kangawa, Minamino, Matsuo, Ueda, Hanaoka, Hirose, and Numa, 1989; Zorzato, Fujii, Otsu, Phillips, Green, Lai, Meissner, and MacLennan, 1990). Transmembrane sequences in the tetramer probably combine to form the membrane-spanning pore of the Ca^{2+} release channel, and cytoplasmic sequences from each subunit appear to interact to form a scaffolding, $29 \times 29 \times 12$ nm in size, that is comprised of 10 or more domains per subunit (Radermacher, Rao, Grassucci, Frank, Timerman, Fleischer, and Wagenknecht, 1994). Regulatory sequences may exist near the transmembrane sequences (Zorzato et al., 1990) or in the cytoplasmic domain (Otsu, Willard, Khanna, Zorzato, Green, and MacLennan, 1990).

The release of Ca^{2+} is the end result of a cascade of events including depolarization of nerve, muscle, and transverse tubular membranes; charge movement associated with the slow Ca^{2+} channel of the transverse tubular membrane (the dihydropyridine receptor) and opening of the Ca^{2+} release channel (Catterall, 1991). Although it is not clear what signals open the channel in the muscle cell, physical interaction between the ryanodine receptor and the DHP receptor is likely to be a component of the mechanism. Ca^{2+} and ATP act synergistically to open the channel in isolated vesicles and Mg^{2+} and calmodulin inhibit channel opening. It is probable that these ligands are also active in vivo.

Human Malignant Hyperthermia

Malignant hyperthermia (MH) is a clinical syndrome in which genetically susceptible individuals respond to potent inhalational anesthetics and depolarizing skeletal muscle relaxants with high fever and skeletal muscle rigidity (Britt, 1991). These symptoms are accompanied by hypermetabolism, leading to hyperventilation, hypoxia, and lactic acidosis. Tachycardia, arrhythmia, and unstable blood pressure are also associated with an MH reaction and these probably result from cellular damage, which brings about electrolyte imbalance and elevation in the serum and urine levels of muscle enzymes and myoglobin. If therapy is not initiated immediately, the patient may die within minutes from ventricular fibrillation, within hours from pulmonary edema or coagulapathy, or within days from neurological damage or obstructive renal failure, resulting largely from the release of muscle proteins into the circulation.

Many patients at risk are identified in advance of anesthesia by knowledge of their relationship to individuals who have had an MH reaction. In these cases, the onset of an MH episode is prevented by including nontriggering anesthetics in the anesthetic routine. During the course of anesthesia, heart rate, body temperature, and end tidal CO_2 production are usually monitored constantly. If any of these should increase so that an MH reaction is suspected, administration of MH-triggering anesthetics is stopped, the patient is hyperventilated with 100% oxygen and the clinical antidote, dantrolene, is administered. These practices have lowered the death rate from MH episodes from over 80% to <7% in western countries in recent years. Neurological, liver or kidney damage, however, still contribute to the morbidity resulting from MH episodes, because damage to muscle cells, leading to leakage of myoplasmic contents, occurs early in the reaction.

Human MH is an autosomal dominant genetic disease. MH reactions do not occur in every case of administration of anesthetics to susceptible individuals, however, and, about half of MH reactions occur in susceptible individuals who have previously had uneventful general anesthetics. Because of the incomplete penetrance of the gene, the difficulty in defining mild reactions and the caution and care now taken by anesthesiologists, it is difficult to determine the actual incidence of MH susceptibility in the general population. Estimates range from ~1 in 15,000 anesthetics in children to ~1 in 50,000 to ~1 in 100,000 anesthetics in adults.

Diagnostic Tests for Malignant Hyperthermia

A major goal of MH research has been to identify MH-susceptible individuals before the administration of anesthetics. If MH susceptibility is known, the use of alternate anesthetics and nondepolarizing muscle relaxants can circumvent the triggering of an MH reaction. Accordingly, the in vitro halothane/caffeine contracture test (CHCT) was developed on the premise that the muscle from MH-susceptible (MHS) individuals might be hypersensitive to these agents and, therefore, might contract in the presence of lower amounts of either caffeine (Kalow, Britt, Terreau, and Haist, 1970) or halothane (Ellis, Harriman, Kyei-Mensah, and Tyrell, 1971) than the muscle from normal individuals.

The CHCT is a valuable clinical test (Larach, 1993). The North American CHCT achieves 92–95% sensitivity and 53–75% specificity for the same tests (Larach, Landis, Shirk, and Diaz, 1992). However, the CHCT is invasive, expensive to perform and has a significant false positive error rate and a very small false negative error rate. While the false positive error rate does not pose a serious problem for clinicians, inaccurate diagnosis creates difficulties for geneticists attempting to link the inheritance of MH susceptibility to inheritance of a specific allele.

Porcine Malignant Hyperthermia

Individuals among herds of lean, heavily muscled swine are susceptible to stress-induced episodes of fever, skeletal muscle rigidity, and hyperventilation (O'Brien, 1987). This syndrome, referred to as the porcine stress syndrome or PSS, is brought on by overheating, exercise, mating, or transportation to market. It occurs in ~1 in 12 animals that are homozygous for the genetic abnormality, but rarely in carriers. Stress-induced deaths in swine occur predominantly with homozygous MH animals. Pigs administered halothane and succinylcholine before surgery have been shown to be susceptible to MH reactions.

The PSS gene is associated with leanness and muscle hypertrophy, and adds to lean, dressed carcass weight (O'Brien, Ball, and MacLennan, 1994). By selecting breeding stock for leanness and heavy muscling, the MH gene is also selected. Recognition that the gene also leads to PSS led to attempts to eliminate the MH gene from swine breeding stock. These efforts were frustrated until we developed diagnostic tests able to detect heterozygous carriers with the accuracy required to eliminate the gene and within acceptable limits of cost (Fujii, Otsu, Zorzato, de Leon, Khanna, Weiler, O'Brien, and MacLennan, 1991).

Physiological Basis of Malignant Hyperthermia

An abnormality in regulation of Ca^{2+} within skeletal muscle could account for all of the symptoms of MH. In particular, contracture may result from the continued presence of Ca^{2+} within the cell and enhanced glycolytic and aerobic metabolism might deplete ATP, glucose, and oxygen, produce excess CO_2, lactic acid and heat, and upset cellular and extracellular ion balances. Because abnormalities in the regulation of the intracellular concentrations of Ca^{2+} that might lead to MH might result from mutations in the Ca^{2+} release channel, others have looked for abnormalities in this function. They found higher rates of Ca^{2+}-induced Ca^{2+} release, particularly at low levels of inducing Ca^{2+}, in preparations from both human (Endo, Yagi, Ishizuka, Horiuti, Koga, and Amaha, 1983) and porcine (Ohnishi, Taylor, and Gronert, 1983) muscle.

Ca^{2+} Release Channel (RYR) Genes

In early studies, we cloned full length cDNAs encoding the rabbit and human skeletal muscle isoforms (RYR1) and the rabbit cardiac isoform (RYR2) of the ryanodine receptor (Otsu et al., 1990; Zorzato et al., 1990). We showed that RYR1 encodes the Ca^{2+} release channel of both slow- and fast-twitch skeletal muscle, whereas RYR2 encodes a second Ca^{2+} release channel that is expressed in cardiac muscle and brain. RYR3 appears to be expressed most abundantly in brain and specific smooth muscles (Hakamata, Nakai, Takeshima, and Imoto, 1992). Thus, RYR1 is the only candidate Ca^{2+} release channel gene for MH.

In our first attempts to associate RYR1 with MH, we localized RYR1 to human chromosome 19q13.1 (MacKenzie, Korneluk, Zorzato, Fujii, Phillips, Iles, Wieringa, Blond, Bailly, Willard, Duff, Worton, and MacLennan, 1990). We then identified a series of restriction-fragment length polymorphisms (RFLPs) in RYR1 that permitted us to study linkage between inheritance of one or more of these RFLPs and inheritance of MH, defined by CHCT (MacLennan, Duff, Zorzato, Fujii, Phillips, Korneluk, Frodis, Britt, and Worton, 1990). Cosegregation was found in 23 meioses in nine families, with no recombinants, leading to a probability of ~ 16,000 to 1 that the two loci are linked. Human markers surrounding human chromosome 19q13.1 were used in an independent study to link MH to the region of human chromosome 19q12–13.2 where RYR1 was localized (McCarthy, Healy, Heffron, Lehane, Deufel, Lehmann-Horn, Faralli, and Johnson, 1990).

Genetic Basis of Porcine Malignant Hyperthermia

In a comparison of RYR1 cDNA sequences from normal (Yorkshire) and MH (Pietrain) pigs, we observed a single deduced amino acid sequence difference (Fujii et al., 1991). The substitution of T for C1843 in the nucleotide sequence also leads to the substitution of Cys for Arg^{615} in the amino acid sequence. We associated this mutation with MH in some 80 animals from five different breeds and then we analyzed linkage in backcrosses between British Landrace N/n and n/n animals (Otsu, Khanna, Archibald, and MacLennan, 1991). In a study of 376 animals, including 338 informative meioses, we observed complete linkage between the presence of the nucleotide 1,843 mutation and phenotypic diagnosis for PSS. Cosegregation of the MH phenotype with the Cys for Arg^{615} substitution led to a lod score (log of the odds favoring linkage) of 102 for a recombination fraction of 0.0.

The same mutation was found in five breeds of pigs, suggesting that it might have originated in a founder animal. Analysis of three polymorphic sites across ~ 150 kbp within the RYR1 gene provided evidence for a common RYR1 haplotype in every MH animal tested, consistent with its origin in a founder animal (Fujii et al., 1991).

The substitution of T for C1843 in the porcine RYR1 gene deletes a HinPI restriction endonuclease site and creates an HgiA1 restriction site. By amplifying a segment of genomic DNA surrounding this site, we developed an accurate diagnostic test on the basis of analysis of the presence or absence of the HinPI or HgiA1 sites (Otsu et al., 1992). Such tests have been readily adapted to large scale commercial testing for the swine industry. They are accurate, noninvasive, and relatively inexpensive, detecting the single mutation found in all breeds. Swine breeders may choose to eliminate all carriers of the PSS gene from apex breeding stocks, or, alternatively, they might decide to take advantage of the beneficial effects of the gene for enhanced lean meat production.

Malignant Hyperthermia Mutations in Humans

The demonstration of linkage between MH and the Arg^{615} to Cys mutation in the porcine RYR1 gene led us to the discovery of the equivalent mutation, Cys for

Arg[614], in human MH families (Gillard, Otsu, Fujii, Khanna, de Leon, Derdemezi, Britt, Duff, Worton, and MacLennan, 1991). The mutation has been found in several MH families worldwide. In most families, it segregates with individuals who have been diagnosed by CHCT as MHS, but in other families it does not. Because the genetic and biochemical evidence supporting the causal nature of this mutation is now so strong, we assume, when linkage of this mutation to MH in humans cannot be demonstrated, that the reason is inaccurate diagnosis of MH through the CHCT.

Eight RYR1 mutations have, so far, been associated with human MH (Gillard et al., 1991; Gillard, Otsu, Fujii, Duff, de Leon, Khanna, Britt, Worton, and MacLennan, 1992; Zhang, Chen, Khanna, de Leon, Phillips, Schappert, Britt, Brownell, and MacLennan, 1993; Quane, Healy, Keating, Manning, Couch, Palmucci, Doriguzzi, Fagerlund, Berg, Ording, Bendixen, Mortier, Linz, Muller, and McCarthy, 1993; Quane, Keating, Manning, Healy, Monsieurs, Heffron, Lehane, Heytons, Krivosic-Harber, Adnet, Ellis, Monnier, Lumardi, and McCarthy, 1994; Quane, Keating, Healy, Manning, Krivosic-Harbey, Monnier, Lunardi, and McCarthy, 1994; Keating, Quane, and Manning, 1995; Table I). These have been discovered either by sequencing of a full-length RYR1 cDNA from an MH proband or by looking for single-strand conformational polymorphisms in amplified segments of RYR1 cDNA or genomic DNA, followed by sequencing. The mutation of Arg[163] to Cys occurs in ~2% of MH families, the mutation of Gly[341] to Arg occurs in ~10% of MH families, the mutation of Arg614 to Cys occurs in ~2% of MH families, and the mutation of Gly2433 to Arg occurs in ~4% of MH families. Thus, over 80% of MH mutations are still to be discovered.

TABLE I
RYR1 Mutations Associated with MH or CCD

Amino Acid Substitution	Nucleotide Substitution	Detection	Association	Reference
Cys for Arg[163]	T for C487	loss of Bst UI	MH, CCD*	Quane et al., 1993
Arg for Gly[248]	A for G742	allele specific PCR	MH	Gillard et al., 1992
Arg for Gly[341]	A for G1021	SSCP	MH	Quane et al., 1994a
Met for Ile[403]	G for C1209	loss of MboI	MH, CCD	Quane et al., 1993
Ser for Tyr[522]	C for A1565	SSCP	MH, CCD	Quane et al., 1994b
Cys for Arg[614]	T for C1840	loss of RsaI	MH	Gillard et al., 1991
Cys for Arg[615] (Pig)	T for C1843	loss of HinPI. gain of HgiAI	MH, PSS	Fujii et al., 1991
Arg for Gly[2433]	A for G7297	gain of Dde1	MH	Keating et al., 1994; Phillips et al., 1994
His for Arg[2434]	A for G7301	loss of HgaI	MH, CCD	Zhang et al., 1993

The search for additional MH mutations is hampered by the size of the cDNA and the gene from which it is derived. Sequencing from genomic DNA will soon be feasible because we are defining exon/intron boundaries and flanking sequences for the RYR1 gene. We have determined that the gene has ~104 exons, two of which are alternatively spliced. Through analysis of phage, YAC and cosmid clones containing the gene, we have shown that the gene covers ~205 kbp (Rouquier, Giorgi, Trask, Bergmann, Phillips, MacLennan, and de Jong, 1993).

Searching for a Second MHS Locus

On the basis of linkage to chromosome 19 and to mutations in RYR1, RYR1 is established as a very strong candidate gene for MH. However, there are cases where diagnosis appears to be accurate and where no linkage between RYR1 and MH can be discerned (e.g., Deufel, Golla, Iles, Meindl, Meitinger, Schindelhauer, DeVries, Pongratz, MacLennan, Johnson, and Lehmann-Horn, 1992). In some laboratories, as few as 35–50% of MH families can be linked to chromosome 19q13.1, suggesting that additional MH gene loci exist (Ball and Johnson, 1993).

Evidence has been presented for a second MHS locus on chromosome 17q21 (Olcklers, Meyers, Meyers, Taylor, Fletcher, Rosenberg, Isaacs, and Levitt, 1992), however, this has not been confirmed (Iles, Segers, Sengers, Monsieurs, Heytens, Halsall, Hopkins, Ellis, Hall-Curran, Stuart, and Weringa, 1993). A single MH family has been linked to a region of chromosome 7 which contains the gene encoding the α-2 subunit of the dihydropyridine receptor (Iles, Lehmann-Horn, Scherer, Tsui, Weghuis, Suijkerbuijk, Heytens, Mikala, Schwartz, Ellis, Stewart, and Wieringa, 1994). To date, the gene has not been sequenced to prove its involvement in MH.

In an effort to determine if any other MHS loci exist, a consortium of scientists forming the genetics section of the European Malignant Hyperthermia Group have screened several three generations, nonchromosome 19 linked families against several hundred microsatellite markers developed by Généthon (Gyapay, Morrissette, Vignal, Deb, Fizames, Mellasseau, Marc, Bernardi, Lathrop, and Weissenbach, 1994), that cover the entire human genome. To date, a single family has been linked to an undisclosed locus with a lod score exceeding 3 (T. Deufel, personal communication).

Central Core Disease

Central core disease is a rare, nonprogressive myopathy characterized by hypotonia and proximal muscle weakness which presents in infancy (Shy and Magee, 1956). Although symptoms may be severe, up to 40% of patients demonstrating central cores may be clinically normal (Shuaib, Paasuke, and Brownell, 1987). Diagnosis is made on the basis of the lack of oxidative enzyme activity in central regions of skeletal muscle cells (Dubowitz and Pearse, 1960), observed upon histological examination of biopsies. Electron microscopic analysis shows disintegration of the contractile apparatus ranging from blurring and streaming of the Z lines to total loss of myofibrillar structure (Brownell, 1988). The sarcoplasmic reticulum and transverse tubular systems are greatly increased in content and are, in general, less well structured. Mitochondria are depleted in the cores, but may be enriched around the surfaces of the cores. Genetic analysis indicates that the disorder is inherited as an autosomal dominant trait with variable penetrance (Mulley, Kozman, Phillips, Gedeon, McCure, Iles, Gregg, Hogan, Couch, Weber, MacLennan, and Haan, 1993). CCD is associated with susceptibility to malignant hyperthermia and linkage of the disease to the long arm of chromosome 19 and to the RYR1 gene was established in large European (Kausch, Lehmann-Horn, Janka, Wieringa, Grimm, and Müller, 1991) and Australian (Mulley, Kozman, Phillips, Gedeon, McCure, Iles, Gregg, Hogan, Couch, Weber, MacLennan, and Haan, 1993) pedigrees.

Analysis of RYR1 cDNA sequences in several CCD families has led to the discovery of four mutations that are linked to CCD as well as to MH (Table I). It is of

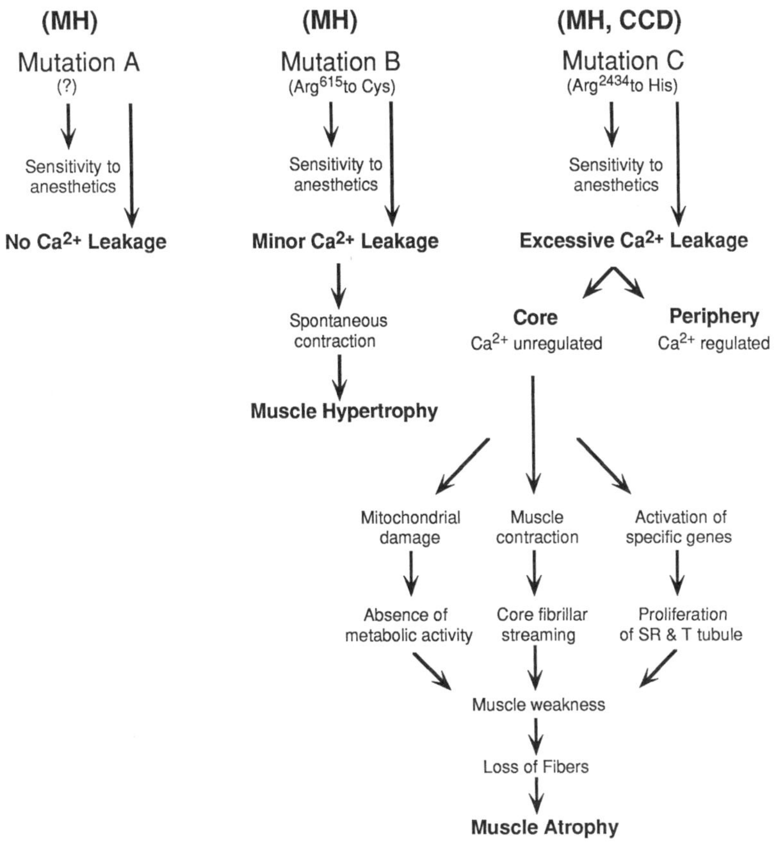

Figure 1. A proposed mechanism for the differential phenotypic effects of different MH and CCD mutations. MH mutations in the ryanodine receptor lead to the common phenotype of sensitivity to anesthetics. Some mutations may also lead to spontaneous Ca^{2+} release sufficient to trigger spontaneous contractions. If this Ca^{2+} trigger were readily regulated, the major phenotypic effect would be spontaneous exercise-induced muscle hypertrophy. The Arg615 to Cys mutation was selected in swine because it leads to increased lean muscle mass. Mutations leading to excessive spontaneous Ca^{2+} release may have no phenotypic effect on the periphery of the cell, but be deleterious to the central core. Ca^{2+} released from the sarcoplasmic reticulum can be regulated by four systems including the organellar sarcoplasmic reticulum and mitochondria and the plasma membrane Ca^{2+} pumps and Na^{+}/Ca^{2+} exchangers. Under normal circumstances, the bulk of the Ca^{2+} is cycled only through the sarcoplasmic reticulum. If enhanced Ca^{2+} release occurred spontaneously, in CCD muscle, the additional Ca^{2+} regulatory systems might be co-opted to regulate Ca^{2+}. The plasma membrane exchangers and pumps would be effective in regulating Ca^{2+} near the periphery, but, in the core, mitochondria may be forced to bear this load, destroying themselves in the process. The degeneration of mitochondria could lead to the degeneration of a central, possibly compartmented, core. The disorganization of the central core might be brought about by higher core levels of Ca^{2+}, which could cause contraction at the core and lead to myofibrillar streaming and membrane disorganization. Elevated Ca^{2+} may stimulate proliferation of internal membrane proteins at the transcriptional level. The phenotypic effects would be the formation of a disorganized, metabolically deficient core which could lead to cell death and muscle atrophy.

interest that six out of eight MH or CCD mutations lie between amino acids 163 and 614 (Table I). The other two mutations, at residues 2433 and 2434, lie at the beginning of a proposed regulatory domain containing potential ATP and calmodulin-binding sites and a phosphorylation site. Such clusters of mutations suggest that these regions of the molecule form regulatory domains in the Ca^{2+} release channel. A second interesting feature of MH mutations discovered so far is the fact that six of the eight involve either loss or gain of an Arg residue (Table I). This suggests that positive changes within the two MH domains are critical to regulatory function.

The discovery of mutations in RYR1 potentially causal of CCD and MH raises interesting questions concerning the pathophysiology of these diseases. It is clear that, in both cases, Ca^{2+} regulation is imbalanced, leading to the contracture and hypermetabolism that characterize MH. In some cases, however, the altered Ca^{2+} regulation leads to muscle hypertrophy, as in the MH pig, while in other cases it leads to disorganization of the contractile proteins in the central core, a proliferation of sarcoplasmic reticulum and transverse tubules and a loss of functional mitochondria as in central core disease. It is possible that these structural alterations arise developmentally and are imposed on the developing fiber by alterations in the physical properties of the Ca^{2+} release channel.

It is also possible that these alterations occur subsequent to the initial formation of a fully functional muscle fiber and are the result of physiological adaptation to functional alterations in the channel that lead to elevated Ca^{2+} levels within the myofibril (Zhang et al., 1993). Myofibrils regulate Ca^{2+} through at least four systems, Ca^{2+} pumps and Na/Ca^{2+} exchangers in the plasma membrane can remove Ca^{2+} from the muscle cell (Carafoli, 1987). Of these, the Ca^{2+} pump has the higher affinity for Ca^{2+}. The sarcoplasmic reticulum is the major regulator of Ca^{2+} within the muscle cell, removing it from the cytoplasm, storing it and releasing it again to initiate muscle contraction. If Ca^{2+} concentrations are elevated, the mitochondria can transport Ca^{2+} to matrix spaces, thereby protecting the cell from Ca^{2+}-induced damage. If the Ca^{2+} release channel were to release excessive amounts of Ca^{2+} within the muscle cell, then the Na^+/Ca^{2+} exchanger and mitochondria might play a more important role in Ca^{2+} regulation in a CCD cell than in a normal cell. Extrusion of excess Ca^{2+} from the cell might, itself, have deleterious effects on the skeletal muscle cell, which is believed to carry out intracellular cycling of a constant level of Ca^{2+} rather than fluxing of Ca^{2+} from external sources.

Pumps and exchangers in the plasma membrane might be more effective in protecting the periphery of the cell than the interior of the cell where the full burden of regulation of excess Ca^{2+} would fall on the sarcoplasmic reticulum and mitochondria. It is possible that mitochondria, which have a high capacity for Ca^{2+} uptake and would, undoubtedly, participate in removal of excess Ca^{2+} from central areas of the cell, might destroy themselves in an effort to protect the cell from Ca^{2+}-induced necrosi (Wrogemann and Pena, 1976). Loss of mitochondria from the center of the cell would, in turn, lead to lower ATP synthesis and might be the underlying cause of the disorganization of the central core, leading to muscle weakness and muscle atrophy. The profusion of sarcoplasmic reticulum and transverse tubules might be induced at the gene level by high local Ca^{2+} concentrations.

Another possibility for the disorganization of the myofibrils in the central core is that high levels of Ca^{2+} in this region might cause localized contracture. This could have the effect of breaking both transverse and longitudinal connections among the fibrils, leading to streaming and blurring of banding patterns in the center of the fibril and to disorganization of the muscle membranes.

It is of interest that the Arg[615] to Cys mutation is associated with muscle hypertrophy in swine while the Arg163 to Cys, Ile403 to Met, Tyr522 to Ser, and Arg2434 to His mutations are associated with variable degrees of muscle atrophy, metabolically inert cores and proximal muscle weakness. If all of these mutations led to poorly regulated Ca^{2+} release into the muscle cell, they could trigger spontaneous muscle contractions. Such spontaneous contractions could lead to the muscle hypertrophy observed in swine. In this case, the system of pumps and exchangers in the plasma membrane and organellar systems of mitochondria and sarcoplasmic reticulum within the cell could remove excess Ca^{2+} from the sarcoplasm without deleterious effects on the muscle cell. The CCD mutations might be more severe, however, leading to damage to the interior of the cell and to loss of mitochondrial function and structural abnormalities in the central core. These, in turn, could lead to muscle weakness and atrophy. Thus, mutations in RYR1 can lead to a spectrum of pathophysiological responses ranging from muscle hypertrophy to muscle atrophy.

Conclusions

Although research has led to a very good understanding of the physiological and genetic basis for malignant hyperthermia in humans and in swine, all of the important goals of MH research have not yet been realized. Perhaps the most important immediate goal is to define all of the genes and all of the mutations in those genes which are causal of human MH. This will provide a firm basis for diagnosis of MH susceptibility for a large fraction of those families in which MH is inherited. A second important goal is to utilize the MH gene in ways that will be of most benefit to the pork industry. A third goal will be to understand structure/function relationships in the ryanodine receptor so that we can better understand the functional consequences of the structural alterations in the Ca^{2+} release channel that lead to its involvement in MH episodes. A fourth goal will be to understand, at the physiological level, how MH and additional abnormalities in muscle cells, such as the formation of central cores, are interrelated and how other myopathies can underlie anesthetic-induced malignant hyperthermia.

Acknowledgements

We thank our many colleagues for advice and discussion in the preparation of this review.

Research grants to D. H. MacLennan, supporting original work from our laboratory, were from the Medical Research Council of Canada (MRCC), the Muscular Dystrophy Association of Canada (MDAC), the Heart and Stroke Foundation of Ontario (HSFO) and the Canadian Genetic Diseases Network of Centers of Excellence. M. S. Phillips is a predoctoral fellow of the HSFO and of the MRCC.

References

Ball, S. P., and K. J. Johnson. 1993. The genetics of malignant hyperthermia. *Journal of Medical Genetics.* 30:89–93.

Britt, B. A. 1991. Malignant hyperthermia: a review. *In* Thermoregulation: Pathology,

Pharmacology, and Therapy. E. Schonbaum and P. Lomax, editors. Pergamon Press Inc., New York. 179–292.

Brownell, A. K. W. 1988. Malignant hyperthermia: relationship to other disease. *British Journal of Anaesthesiology.* 60:303–308.

Carafoli, E. 1987. Intracellular calcium homeostasis. *Annual Review of Biochemistry.* 56:395–433.

Catterall, W. A. 1991. Excitation-contraction coupling in vertebrate skeletal muscle: a tale of two calcium channels. *Cell.* 64:871–874.

Deufel, T., A. Golla, D. Iles, A. Meindl, T. Meitinger, D. Schindelhauer, A. DeVries, D. Pongratz, D. H. MacLennan, K. J. Johnson, and F. Lehmann-Horn. 1992. Evidence for genetic heterogeneity of malignant hyperthermia susceptibility. *American Journal of Human Genetics.* 50:1151–1161.

Dubowitz, V., and A. G. E. Pearse. 1960. Oxidative enzymes and phosphorylase in central-core disease of muscle. *The Lancet*. 23–24.

Ellis, F. R., D. G. F. Harriman, K. Kyei-Mensah, and J. H.Tyrell. 1971. Halothane-induced muscle contracture as a cause of hyperpyrexia. *British Journal of Anaesthesiology.* 43:721.

Endo, M., S. Yagi, T. Ishizuka, K. Horiuti, Y. Koga, and K. Amaha. 1983. Changes in the Ca-induced Ca release mechanism in sarcoplasmic reticulum from a patient with malignant hyperthermia. *Biomedical Research.* 4:83–92.

Fujii, J., K. Otsu, F. Zorzato, S. deLeon, V. K. Khanna, J. Weiler, P. J. O'Brien, and D. H. MacLennan. 1991. Identification of a mutation in porcine ryanodine receptor associated with malignant hyperthermia. *Science.* 253:448–451.

Gillard, E. F., K. Otsu, J. Fujii, C. L. Duff, S. de Leon, V. K. Khanna, B. A. Britt, R. G. Worton, and D. H. MacLennan. 1992. Polymorphisms and deduced amino acid substitutions in the coding sequence of the ryanodine receptor (RYR1) gene in individuals with malignant hyperthermia. *Genomics.* 13:1247–1254.

Gillard, E. F., K. Otsu, J. Fujii, V. K. Khanna, S. de Leon, J. Derdemezi, B. A. Britt, C. L. Duff, R. G. Worton, and D. H. MacLennan. 1991. A substitution of cysteine for arginine-614 in the ryanodine receptor is potentially causative of human malignant hyperthermia. *Genomics.* 11:751–755.

Gyapay, G., J. Morrissette, A. Vignal, C. Deb, C. Fizames, P. Mellasseau, S. Marc, G. Bernardi, M. Lathrop, and J. Weissenbach. 1994. The 1993–94 Généthon human linkage map. *Nature Genetics*. 7:246–339.

Hakamata, Y., J. Nakai, H. Takeshima, and K. Imoto. 1992. Primary structure and distribution of a novel ryanodine receptor/calcium release channel from rabbit brain. *FEBS Letters.* 312:229–235.

Iles, D. E., B. Segers, R. C. A. Sengers, K. Monsieurs, L. Heytens, P. J. Halsall, P. M. Hopkins, F. R. Ellis, J. L. Hall-Curran, A. D. Stuart, and B. Wieringa. 1993. Genetic mapping of the beta 1 and gamma subunits of the human skeletal muscle L-type voltage dependent calcium channel on chromosome 17q and exclusion as a candidate gene for malignant hyperthermia susceptibility. *Human Molecular Genetics.* 2:863–868.

Iles, D. E., F. Lehmann-Horn, S. W. Scherer, L. C. Tsui, D. O. Weghuis, R. F. Suijkerbuijk, L. Heytens, G. Mikala, A. Schwartz, F. R. Ellis, A. D. Stewart, and B. Wieringa. 1994. Localization of the gene encoding the alpha2/d-subunits of the L-type voltage-dependent calcium channel to chromosome 7q and analysis of the segregation of flanking markers in malignant hyperthermia susceptible families. *Human Molecular Genetics.* 3:969–975.

Kalow, W., B. A. Britt, M. E. Terreau, and C. Haist. 1970. Metabolic error of muscle metabolism after recovery from malignant hyperthermia. *The Lancet.* ii:895–898.

Kausch, K., F. Lehmann-Horn, M. Janka, B. Wieringa, T. Grimm, and C. R. Müller. 1991. Evidence for linkage of the central core disease locus to the proximal long arm of human chromosome 19. *Genomics.* 10:765–769

Keating, K. E., K. A. Quane, and B. M. Manning. 1994. Detection of a novel RYR1 mutation in four malignant hyperthermia pedigrees. *Human Molecular Genetics.* 3:1855–1858.

Larach, M. G. 1993. Should we use muscle biopsy to diagnose malignant hyperthermia susceptibility? *Anesthesiology.* 79:1–4.

Larach, M. G., J. R. Landis, B. S. Shirk, M. Diaz, and The North American Malignant Hyperthermia Registry. 1992. Prediction of malignant hyperthermia susceptibility in man: improving sensitivity of the caffeine halothane contracture test. *Anesthesiology.* 77:A1052. (Abstr.)

MacKenzie, A. E., R. G. Korneluk, F. Zorzato, J. Fujii, M. Phillips, D. Iles, B. Wieringa, S. Le Blond, J. Bailly, H. F. Willard, C. Duff, R. G. Worton, and D. H. MacLennan. 1990. The human ryanodine receptor gene: its mapping to 19q13.1, placement in a chromosome 19 linkage group and exclusion as the gene causing myotonic dystrophy. *American Journal of Human Genetics.* 46:1082–1089.

MacLennan, D. H., C. Duff, F. Zorzato, J. Fujii, M. Phillips, R. G. Korneluk, W. Frodis, B. A. Britt, and R. G. Worton. 1990. Ryanodine receptor gene is a candidate for predisposition to malignant hyperthermia. *Nature.* 343:559–561.

McCarthy, T. V., J. M. S. Healy, J. J. A. Heffron, M. Lehane, T. Deufel, F. Lehmann-Horn, M. Faralli, and K. Johnson. 1990. Localization of the malignant hyperthermia susceptibility locus to human chromosome 19q12–13.2. *Nature.* 343:562–564.

Mulley, J. C., H. M. Kozman, H. A. Phillips, A. K. Gedeon, J. A. McCure, D. E. Iles, R. G. Gregg, K. Hogan, F. J. Couch, J. L. Weber, D. H. MacLennan, and E. A. Haan. 1993. Refined genetic localization for central core disease. *American Journal of Human Genetics.* 52:398–405

O'Brien, P. J. 1987. Etiopathogenetic defect of malignant hyperthermia: hypersensitive calcium-release channel of skeletal muscle sarcoplasmic reticulum. *Veterinary Research Communication.* 11:527–559.

O'Brien, P. J., R. O. Ball, and D. H. MacLennan. 1994. Effects of heterozygosity for the mutation causing porcine stress syndrome on carcass quality and live performance characteristics. *In* Proceedings of the 13th International Pig Veterinary Society Congress, Bangkok. 481.

Ohnishi, S. T., S. Taylor, and G. A. Gronert. 1983. Calcium-induced Ca^{2+} release from sarcoplasmic reticulum of pigs susceptible to malignant hyperthermia. The effects of halothane and dantrolene. *FEBS Letters.* 161:103–107.

Olckers, A., D. A. Meyers, S. Meyers, E. W. Taylor, J. E. Fletcher, H. Rosenberg, H. Isaacs, and R. D. Levitt. 1992. Adult muscle sodium channel α–subunit is a gene candidate for malignant hyperthermia susceptibility. *Genomics.* 14:829–831.

Otsu, K., H. F. Willard, V. K. Khanna, F. Zorzato, N. M. Green, and D. H. MacLennan. 1990. Molecular cloning of cDNA encoding the Ca^{2+} release channel (ryanodine receptor) of rabbit cardiac muscle sarcoplasmic reticulum. *Journal of Biological Chemistry.* 265:13472–13483.

Otsu, K., M. S. Phillips, V. K. Khanna, S. de Leon, and D. H. MacLennan. 1992. Refinement of diagnostic assays for a probable causal mutation for porcine and human malignant hyperthermia. *Genomics.* 13:835–837.

Otsu, K., V. K. Khanna, A. L. Archibald, and D. H. MacLennan. 1991. Co-segregation of porcine malignant hyperthermia and a probable causal mutation in the skeletal muscle ryanodine receptor gene in backcross families. *Genomics.* 11:744–750.

Phillips, M. S., V. K. Khanna, S. de Leon, W. Frodis, B. A. Britt, and D. H. MacLennan. 1994. The substitution of Arg for Gly2433 in the human skeletal muscle ryanodine receptor is associated with malignant hyperthermia. *Human Molecular Genetics*. 3:2181–2186.

Quane, K. A., J. M. S. Healy, K. E. Keating, B. M. Manning, F. J. Couch, L. M. Palmucci, C. Doriguzzi, T. H. Fagerlund, K. Berg, H. Ording, D. Bendixen, W. Mortier, U. Linz, C. R. Muller, and T. V. McCarthey. 1993. Mutations in the ryanodine receptor gene in central core disease and malignant hyperthermia. *Nature Genetics*. 5:51–55.

Quane, K. A., K. E. Keating, B. M. Manning, J. M. S. Healy, K. Monsieurs, J. J. A. Heffron, M. Lehane, L. Heytens, R. Krivosic-Harber, P. Adnet, F. R. Ellis, N. Monnier, J. Lumardi, and T. V. McCarthy. 1994. Detection of a novel common mutation in the ryanodine receptor gene in malignant hyperthermia: implications for diagnosis and heterogeneity studies. *Human Molecular Genetics.* 3:471–476.

Quane, K. A., K. E. Keating, J. M. S. Healy, B. M. Manning, R. Krivosic-Harbey, I. Krivosic, N. Monnier, J. Lunardi, and T. V. McCarthy. 1994 Mutation screening of the RYR1 gene in malignant hyperthermia: detection of a novel Tyr to Ser mutation in a pedigree with associated central cores. *Genomics*. 23:236–239.

Radermacher, M., V. Rao, R. Grassucci, J. Frank, A. Timerman, S. Fleischer, and T. Wagenknecht. 1994. Cryo-electron microscopy and three-dimensional reconstruction of the calcium release channel/ryanodine receptor from skeletal muscle. *Journal of Cell Biology.* 127:411–423.

Rouquier, S., D. Giorgi, B. Trask, A. Bergmann, M. S. Phillips, D. H. MacLennan, and P. de Jong, 1993. A cosmid and yeast artificial chromosome contig containing the complete ryanodine receptor (RYR1) gene. *Genomics*. 17:330–340.

Shuaib, A., R. T. Paasuke, and K. W. Brownell. 1987. Central core disease: clinical features in 13 patients. *Medicine.* 66:389–396.

Shy, G. M., and K. R. Magee. 1956. A new congenital non-progressive myopathy. *Brain.* 79:610–621.

Smith, J. S., R. Coronado, and G. Meissner. 1985. Sarcoplasmic reticulum contains adenine nucleotide activated calcium channels. *Nature.* 316:446–449.

Takeshima, H., S. Nishimura, T. Matsumoto, H. Ishida, K. Kangawa, N. Minamino, H. Matsuo, M. Ueda, M. Hanaoka, T. Hirose, and S. Numa. 1989. Primary structure and expression from complementary DNA of skeletal muscle ryanodine receptor. *Nature.* 339:439–445.

Wagenknecht, T., R. Grassucci, J. Frank, A. Saito, M. Inui, and S. Fleischer. 1989. Three-dimensional architecture of the calcium channel/foot structure of sarcoplasmic reticulum. *Nature.* 338:167–170.

Wrogemann, K., and S. D. J. Pena. 1976. Mitochondrial calcium overload: a general mechanism for cell necrosis in muscle diseases. *The Lancet.* 1:672–673.

Zhang, Y., H. S. Chen, V. K. Khanna, S. de Leon, M. S. Phillips, K. Schappert, B. A. Britt, A. K. W. Brownell, and D. H. MacLennan. 1993. Identification of a mutation in human ryanodine receptor associated with central core disease. *Nature Genetics.* 5:61–65.

Zorzato, F., J. Fujii, K. Otsu, M. Phillips, N. M. Green, F. A. Lai, G. Meissner, and D. H. MacLennan. 1990. Molecular cloning of cDNA encoding human and rabbit forms of the release channel (ryanodine receptor) of skeletal muscle sarcoplasmic reticulum. *Journal of Biological Chemistry.* 265:2244–2256.

Altered Calcium Currents in Human Hypokalemic Periodic Paralysis Myotubes Expressing Mutant L-type Calcium Channels

Frank Lehmann-Horn,* Istvan Sipos,*‖ Karin Jurkat-Rott,* Roland Heine,* Heinrich Brinkmeier,‡ Bertrand Fontaine,§ Laszlo Kovacs,‖ and Werner Melzer*

**Departments of Applied and ‡General Physiology, University of Ulm, D-89081 Ulm, Germany; §INSERM U134, Fédération de Neurologie, Hôpital de la Salpêtrière, 75013 Paris, France; and ‖Department of Physiology, University Medical School of Debrecen, H-4012 Debrecen, Hungary*

In a genome-wide search, linkage of hypokalemic periodic paralysis (HypoPP), a muscle disease with autosomal dominant inheritance, to chromosome 1q31-32 and cosegregation with the gene encoding the L-type calcium channel/DHP receptor $\alpha 1$ subunit has been reported (Fontaine et al., 1994). Here we show the extended haplotypes of a large HypoPP family who made the detection of the gene product possible. Sequencing of cDNA synthesized from RNA isolated from muscle specimens of two affected family members revealed a G-to-A transition of nucleotide 3716. This base exchange predicts a substitution of histidine for arginine 1239 located in segment IVS4 of the channel protein. By restriction fragment analysis, the mutation was detected in the genomic DNA of all affected family members. Myotubes cultured from the muscle specimens also revealed the mutation suggesting the expression of mutant L-type calcium channel/DHP receptors. Whole-cell recordings of 20 such myotubes showed a strong reduction of the DHP sensitive, slowly activating and inactivating L-type current density to 30% of the current in normal controls. A rapidly activating and inactivating current component (third-type), which is distinct from the also occurring T-type current, was increased. We conclude that HypoPP is a disease of the skeletal muscle DHP receptor. The point mutation in repeat IV of the protein may have a similar effect as drugs which downregulate the channel activity by binding to this domain.

Introduction

Dihydropyridine (DHP) receptors are located in the transverse tubular system of skeletal muscle fibers and consist of five subunits: α_1, α_2/δ, β, and γ (Catterall, 1988). The α_1 subunit (Tanabe, Takeshima, Mikami, Flockerzi, Takahashi, Kangawa, Kojima, Matsuo, Hirose, and Numa, 1987) contains the putative voltage sensing structures (the S4 segments in the four homologous repeats), receptors for calcium channel agonists and antagonists such as dihydropyridines and phenylalkamines, as well as the calcium conducting pore (Tanabe, Mikami, Niidome, Numa, Adams, and Beam, 1993; Mori et al., 1993; Hofmann, Biel, and Flockerzi, 1994). The receptor is thought to fulfill a dual function as calcium channel and as voltage sensor for the control of calcium release from the sarcoplasmic reticulum. Both functions are eliminated in mouse skeletal muscle fibers homozygous for the mdg mutation (muscular dysgenesis) which disables the α_1 subunit of the L-type calcium channel/DHP receptor (Beam et al., 1986; Chaudhari, 1992). They could be recovered by injecting the cDNA of the rabbit α_1 subunit (Tanabe, Beam, Powell, and Numa, 1988). The mdg mouse was the only example so far of an abnormal phenotype linked to a mutation in a voltage-gated calcium channel.

Recently, evidence was presented that the hereditary human muscle disease hypokalemic periodic paralysis (HypoPP) is linked to the gene encoding the L-type calcium channel/DHP receptor α_1 subunit of skeletal muscle (Fontaine et al., 1994; Jurkat-Rott et al., 1994) which has been localized to region q32.1–q32.2 on chromosome 1 (Drouet, Garcia, Simon-Chazottes, Mattei, Guénet, Schwartz, Varadi, and Pinçon-Raymond, 1993). The linkage data induced successful searches for mutations in this gene predicting arginine to histidine substitutions in IIS4 and IVS4 and in addition a substitution of glycine for the same arginine in IVS4 (Jurkat-Rott et al., 1994; Ptácek et al., 1994).

HypoPP is the most common of the primary periodic paralyses. It is an autosomal dominant disease characterized by attacks of flaccid weakness which are provoked by excessive intake of carbohydrates, rest after strenuous exercise or mental stress. A stimulation of the sodium-potassium pump by insuline is assumed to be the mechanism by which potassium ions are transported from the extracellular into the intracellular compartment causing hypokalemia (for review see Lehmann-Horn, Engel, Rüdel, and Ricker, 1994). Next to a fall of serum potassium, other factors influencing frequency and severity of clinical symptoms might be other hormones, as onset is usually during puberty, as penetrance in women is incomplete, as attacks become predominant during pregnancy, and as adrenaline is a specific triggering agent.

Here we report more evidence for tight genetic linkage between HypoPP in a large pedigree and the gene of the L-type calcium channel/DHP receptor α_1 subunit. Furthermore, we demonstrate the presence of a IVS4 mutation in all affected members. For the study of the functional consequences of the mutation on the gene product we measured calcium currents on myotubes derived from two patients of this family as partially described by Sipos, Szücs, Struk, Lehmann-Horn, and Melzer (1994).

Material and Methods

Genomic DNA was extracted from anticoagulated blood of all individuals with their informed consent. Muscle specimens were obtained from two patients and 15 individuals who had undergone muscle biopsy for exclusion of malignant hyperthermia susceptibility; these specimens served as controls if susceptibility was excluded. All procedures were in accordance with the Helsinki convention and were approved by the Ethical Committee of the University of Ulm.

Genetic Linkage

Genotyping of all microsatellites was performed by the polymerase chain reaction (PCR) according to Généthon standard protocols. Dinucleotide repeats (Gyapay et al., 1994) and three additional microsatellites developed at Généthon were used:

AFM136xa7; AFM337xd5; AFM312yb5 (Jurkat-Rott et al., 1994). The likelihood of the order of the loci, genetic distances, and localization of the DHP-receptor were established with odds over 10^3:1 after genotyping the microsatellites in eight C.E.P.H. families using the program ILINK of the LINKAGE package (version 5.1). Recombination fractions were converted to map distances using the Haldane mapping function.

Molecular Biology

As sequencing of cDNA had shown a G-to-A transition at position 3716 of the human α_1 subunit, a method was developed for screening of the genomic DNA of the family members. Short fragments (length of PCR product 94 bp) of genomic DNA were amplified by PCR with primers derived from the human cDNA sequence (Hogan, K., P. Powers, and R. Gregg, 1994): as forward primer 5′-CGCATCTCCAGC-GCCTTCTTC-3′ and 5′ACGTCCACAGGAGGGTTCGCACT-3′ as reverse primer.

The reaction mixture with a final volume of 100 μl contained: 50 ng DNA, 50 pmol of each PCR primer, 50 μM of each deoxynucleotide triphosphate, 10 mM Tris (pH 8.3), 50 mM KCl, 1.5 mM $MgCl_2$ and 1.5 U of Taq polymerase. Amplification conditions: 10 min at 96°C, followed by 30 cycles of 94°C for 30 s, 66°C for 45 s, and 72°C for 1 min. After precipitation of the total volume of the PCR product in 300 μl ethanol and redissolving in 30 μl distilled water, a digestion with 1 U of NlaIII (New England Biolabs, Beverly, MA) was performed at 37°C for 8 h. The reaction was stopped with 3 μl of blue sucrose (30% sucrose, 50 mM EDTA, 0.25% bromophenol blue, 0.1% SDS). 6 μl of the product were loaded on a 15% acrylamide gel and run at 300 V for 3–4 h in TBE buffer. After electrophoresis, the gels were stained with 0.5 μg/ml ethidium bromide. Direct sequencing was performed as earlier described (Heine, Pika, and Lehmann-Horn, 1993).

Cell Culture

Biopsies were obtained from the vastus lateralis muscle. The procedure of growing myotubes from human satellite cells followed closely the description by Brinkmeier, Mutz, Seewald, Melzner, and Rüdel (1993). Briefly, the biopsy material was dissociated enzymatically at 37°C in PBS solution (Biochrom) containing collagenase (250 U/ml, Type II, Sigma Chemical Co., St. Louis, MO) and bactotrypsin (3%, Difco Laboratories, Inc., Detroit, MI). The reaction was stopped with Hank's solution containing 10% FCS (fetal calf serum). After filtering and centrifugation (100 *g*, 10 min) the pellet was resuspended in a culture medium consisting of a mixture (1:1) of Ham's F-12 and CMRL medium (Biochrom, Berlin, Germany) containing 5% FCS, 5% HS (both GIBCO-BRL, Gaithersburg, MD), 2.5 mg/ml glucose, 0.3 mg/ml glutamine (Biochrom) and 1.2 mg/ml $NaHCO_3$ and kept in a 5% CO_2 atmosphere. After 1–2 d, the serum content of the culture medium was reduced to 2% FCS and 2% HS. Fusion of myotubes sufficient for electrophysiological studies was observed after 10–14 d.

Screening of the RNA of Cultured Cells

RNA was isolated from the cultured cells using TRIzol (GIBCO-BRL) and reverse transcriptase PCR with the screening primers mentioned above was performed according to (Jurkat-Rott et al., 1994). PCR products were tested for the mutation as described above in Molecular Biology.

Electrophysiology

Whole-cell recordings were performed by use of an EPC-7 patch clamp amplifier (List Biological Laboratories, Inc., Campbell, CA). The currents were sampled at 2–10 kHz using commercial data acquisition hard and software (TL1 and Pclamp 5.51, Axon Instruments, Inc., Foster City, CA) on an IBM AT486 compatible microcomputer. The linear capacitance of the myotubes was determined by the integral of the transient current divided by the corresponding voltage step amplitude (+5 mV). The series resistance was calculated by the ratio of the time constant of the transient current decay and the capacitance. Statistics were performed by use of the two-tailed *t* test. Values are given as mean ± SD.

Calcium currents were studied in a solution in which the major cations, potassium and sodium, were replaced by ions incapable of permeating the membrane of the myotubes. The bathing solution contained (in millimolar): TEA-Cl 120, $CaCl_2$ 10, $MgCl_2$ 1, HEPES 10, Glucose 5, TTX 0.02, EGTA 0.1; pH at 7.4). The patch pipettes were filled with CsCl 130, $MgCl_2$ 0.5, HEPES 10, EGTA 1, Mg-ATP 5, creatine phosphate 5; pH at 7.2. All measurements were performed at room temperature.

Results

HypoPP Family Pedigree, Haplotypes, and Genetic Map

For a more precise mapping of the HypoPP locus and to yield a higher lod score, we extended the linkage study for our family (already partially published as family B by Fontaine et al. [1994] and Jurkat-Rott et al. [1994]) by inclusion of additional family members and the use of three AFM microsatellites located between D1S413 and D1S510. Because an affected member of our family is recombinant for both AFM312yb5 and AFM136xa7 but is not recombinant for the other markers, we deduced that these markers are located telomerically to AFM337xd5 (Fig. 1). Because an affected member of another pedigree (family A in Jurkat-Rott et al. [1994]) is recombinant for both D1S413 and AFM337xd5 (not shown), the respective position of AFM337xd5 and AFM136xa7 is confirmed. Due to the uninformativeness of D1S306 for the two crucial recombinants, the HypoPP locus could not be placed relative to this microsatellite. Therefore, the HypoPP locus is flanked by AFM337xd5 and AFM136xa7 (Fig. 2) which are separated by a genetic distance of 0 cM as calculated in the eight C.E.P.H. families used to type the Généthon markers for chromosome 1. The highest two-point LOD scores at a recombination fraction of zero were found for AFM337xd5 (Z_{max} = 5.26).

Search for the Mutation in cDNA

Total RNA was isolated from muscle specimens obtained from one patient of our family and from four controls. RNA was reverse transcribed and regions of the CACNL1A3 cDNA were amplified by use of PCR primers derived from human cDNA sequence (Hogan, Powers, and Gregg, 1994). Amplified DNA fragments obtained by asymmetrical PCR were purified and directly sequenced. Of the full-length cDNA (~5,600 bp), 4,100 bp encoding the four (highly conserved) domains were sequenced. We identified a G-to-A transition of nucleotide 3716 which results in an arginine to histidine substitution at position 1239 (Fig. 3*A*). This amino

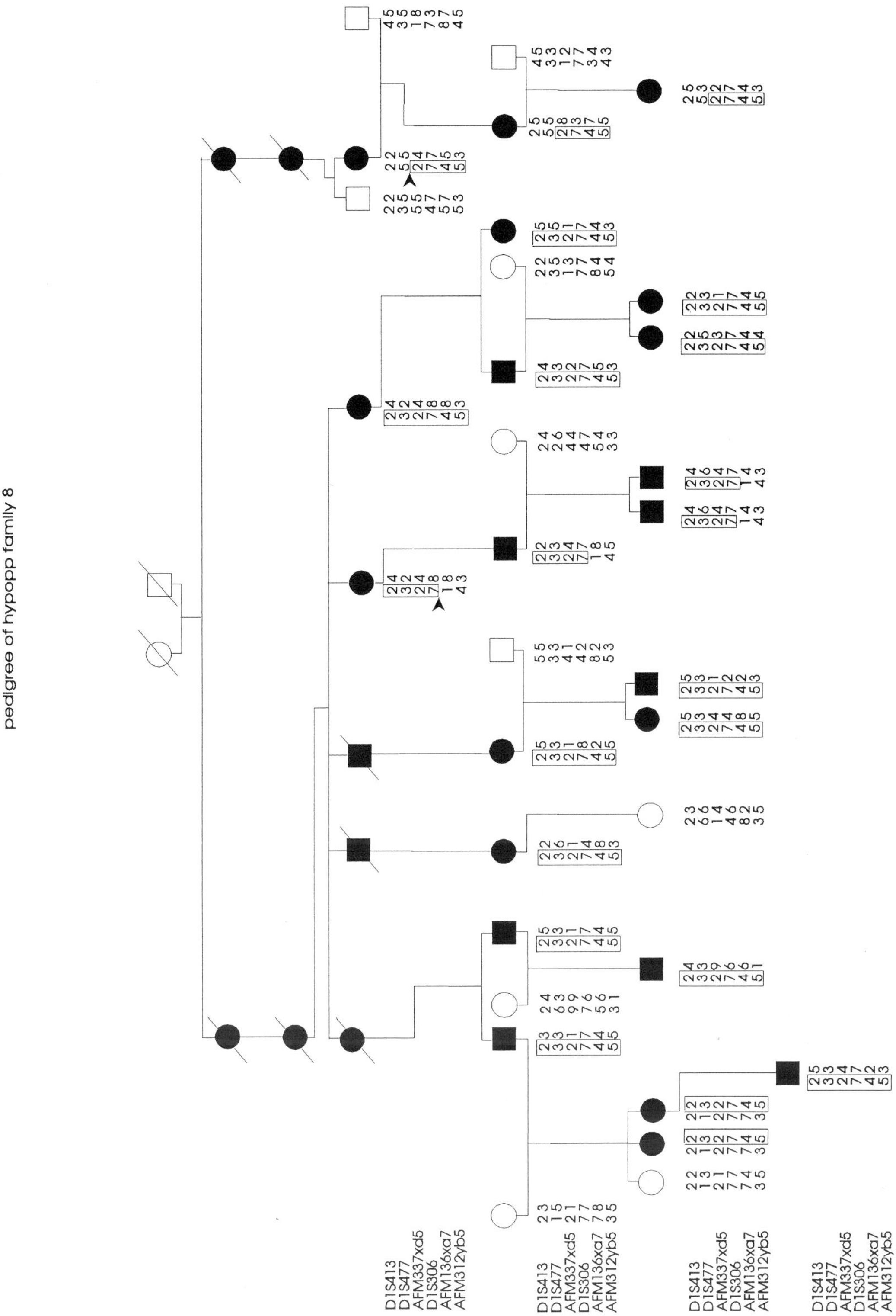

Figure 1. HypoPP family pedigree and haplotypes. (*Filled symbols*) Patients; (*open symbols*) uneffected individuals. The haplotypes segregating with the disease is boxed. (*Arrow heads*) Recombination events.

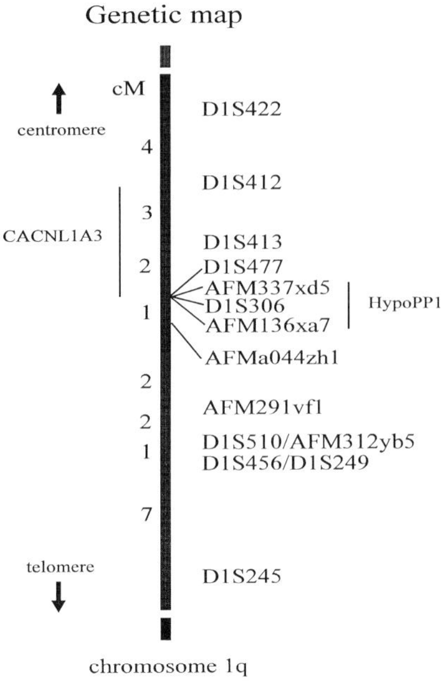

Figure 2. Genetic map of region q32 of chromosome 1 including the localization of the HypoPP locus between AFM337xd5 and AFM136xa7. The locus of CACNL1A3 (which could not be localized more precisely than between D1S412 and the cluster of D1S477/AFM337xd5/D1S306/AFM136xa7 due to the uninformativeness of the intragenic markers available) is also indicated. Note that the overlapping region is equivalent to the HypoPP locus and is likely to contain at least part of CACNL1A3.

acid is located in repeat IV within an α helix containing a positively charged amino acid at every third position, a putative voltage sensor of the channel protein.

Presence of the Mutation in Genomic DNA and RNA of Myotubes

Introduction of a restriction site by the base exchange and design of adequate exon primers, made it possible to screen genomic DNA in all family members. The mutation segregated perfectly with the disease (Fig. 3 *B*) and was not present in DNA of 100 control subjects (200 chromosomes). In addition to the normal sequence, the mutation was also found in the RNA isolated from myotubes derived from the two patients biopsied (Fig. 3 *C*). Because the RNA isolation occurred at the same culture stage as the electrophysiogical studies, the presence of both the mutated and the normal channel protein in the myotubes could be expected.

Figure 3. (*A*) Schematic diagram of the DHP-receptor α_1 subunit consisting of four regions of internal homology, so-called repeats, connected by intracellular loops. Each repeat contains six hydrophobic segments (S1–S6), putative transmembrane helices. An interlinker is found between segments S5 and S6 of each repeat, consisting of an extracellular loop and a sequence which reemerges into the membrane lining the channel pore. Segment IVS4 containing positive charges at each third position is enlarged in the inset showing the ariginine to histidine mutation found in all affected family members. (*B*) Partial pedigree of the HypoPP family with corresponding polyacrylamide gel displaying PCR-amplified genomic DNA fragments after digestion with NlaIII and staining with ethidium bromide. PCR products of unaffected individuals show complete digestion: two bands of 55 and 39 bp; patients' DNA shows an additional band of 34 bp resulting from the mutated PCR product due to introduction of a new restriction site in the mutant DNA. (*C*) Presence of the mutation in myotubes. For details see Methods and Fig. 3 *B*.

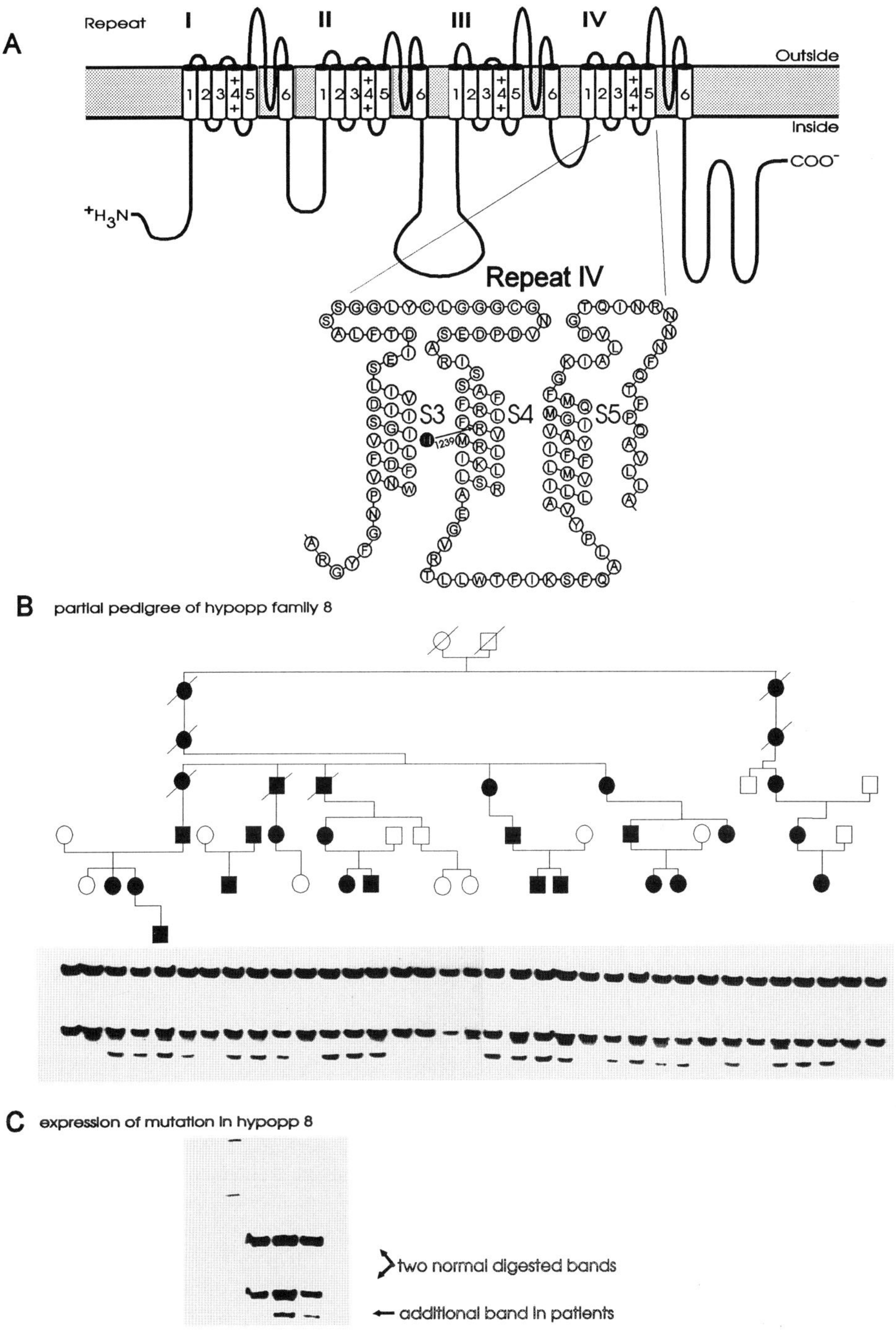
A
Repeat
I
II
III
IV
Outside
Inside
+H3N
COO−
Repeat IV
S3
S4
S5
1239
B partial pedigree of hypopp family 8
C expression of mutation in hypopp 8
two normal digested bands
additional band in patients

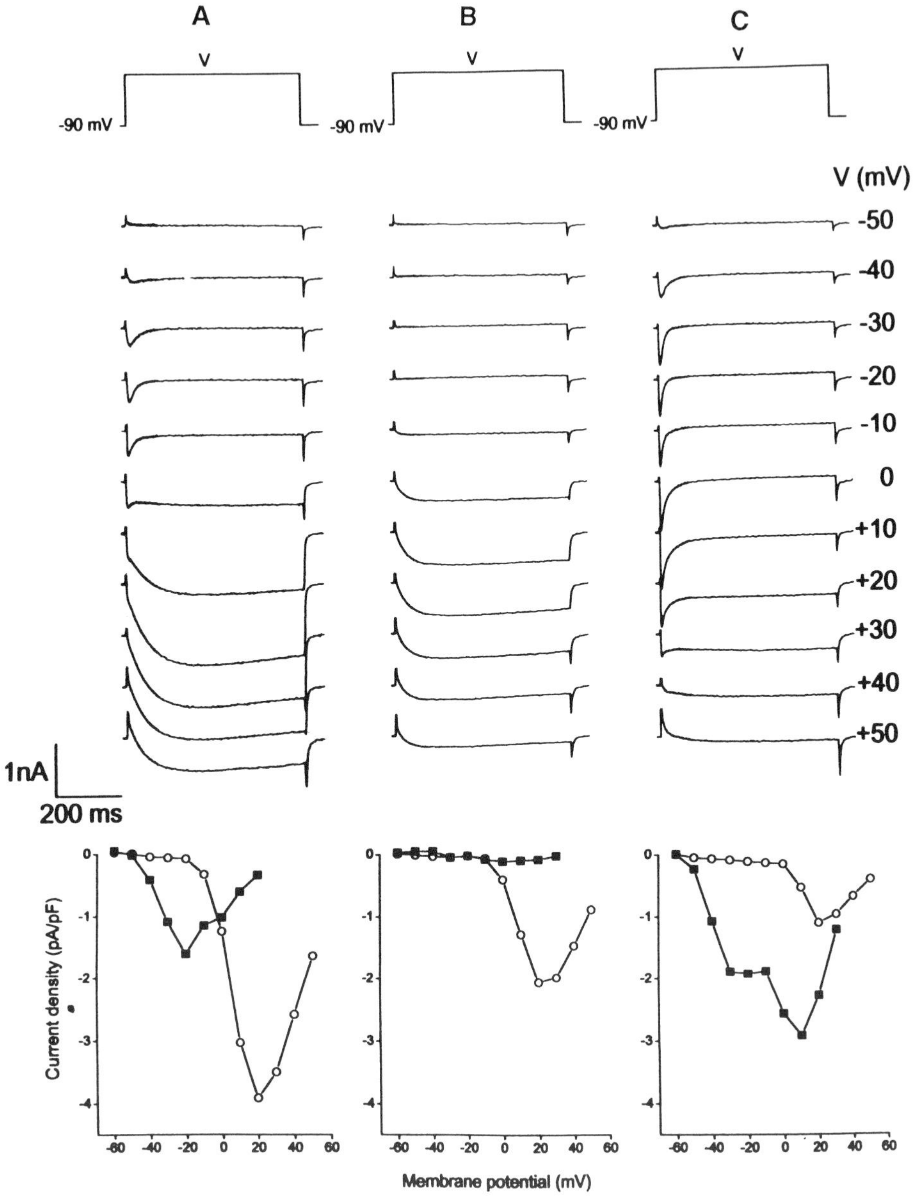

Figure 4. Whole-cell currents recorded on human myotubes cultured from muscle specimens obtained from normal controls (*top*) and corresponding current-voltage relations showing the peak current normalized by the linear capacitance of the given myotube (*bottom;* fast currents: *filled symbols;* slow currents: *open symbols*). The myotubes revealed a rapidly activating and inactivating calcium current with a voltage threshold at ~ −50 mV (T-type current; *A*) and a slowly activating and inactivating (L-type; *A* and *B*) current. Some myotubes showed a second type of fast current exhibiting maximum inward current at more positive potential (third type; *C*).

Voltage-gated Calcium Currents in Normal Human Myotubes

The majority of 57% of the 47 cells studied exhibited a rapidly activating and inactivating calcium current component with a voltage threshold at ~ −50 mV (T-type current) in addition to the slow (L-type) current which started to activate at ~ −20 mV (Fig. 4 *A*). In the remaining myotubes, the fast current was missing and only the L-type current could be activated (Fig. 4 *B*). In 34% of the total number of cells, a second type of fast current was recorded which revealed kinetics similar to the T-type but exhibited a maximum inward current at ~30 mV more positive potential (third-type according to Rivet, Cognard, Imbert, Rideau, Duport, and Raymond, 1992). To show this component clearly, one cell was selected which had a large amplitude of the third-type current and an unusually small L-type current (Fig. 4 *C*).

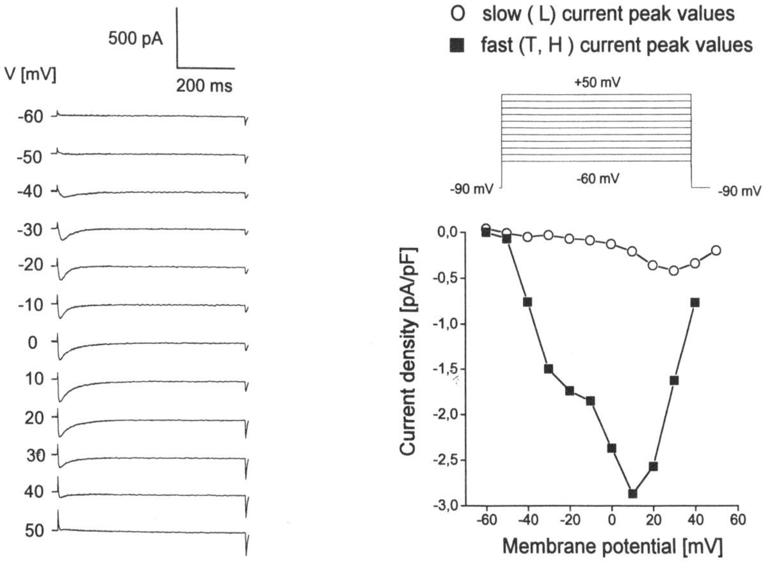

Figure 5. Whole-cell currents recorded on human myotubes cultured from muscle specimens obtained from a patient (*left*) and a representative current-voltage relationships which shows the peak current density (*right; fast currents: filled symbols;* slow currents: *open symbols*).

Average current-voltage relationships showed that the third-type current is too small so that it could not form a distinct peak of the relation combining both fast current types (not shown). The average current density of the L-type current amounted to −1.41 ± 0.71 pA/pF when activated by a pulse to +20 mV.

Voltage-gated Calcium Currents in Human Myotubes Expressing the Mutation

In the 20 myotubes expressing the IVS4 mutation, the L-type current density was drastically reduced to 30% of the control value: the peak value was −0.42 ± 0.25 pA/pF at +20 mV. Original traces and the determined current-voltage relationship of a representative HypoPP myotube is shown in Fig. 5. The percentage of cells expressing the third-type current was considerably increased (from 34 to 75%). Thus, we noted a significant increase in the average peak value of this fast current which exhibited its maximum at 0 to +10 mV. The differences between control and HypoPP myotubes were statistically significant in the 0–50 mV range for the L-type and in the 10–30 mV range for the third-type current (P = 0.02).

Because the reduction of the L-type current could have been due to a voltage-dependent inactivation to more negative potentials, which might have lowered channel availability already at the holding potential of −90 mV, we applied prepulses which hyperpolarized the membrane for 20 s to −120 mV. This did not lead to a restoration of the current amplitude and thus excluded this possible explanation.

Discussion

CACNL1A3 co-segregates with the HypoPP locus without any recombinations, and the detected G3716A base exchange fulfills all criteria of a causal mutation such as: (*a*) absence in a large number of controls (100 individuals with no known neuromuscular disease); (*b*) segregation with the clinical status of all family members examined; (*c*) presence in a gene primarily or exclusively expressed in the affected cells (the skeletal muscle); (*d*) location in a functionally important, highly conserved gene region (a positive charge within IVS4); and (*e*) change of the function of the gene product (reduced L-type current observed in the HypoPP myotubes).

The results on normal human myotubes confirm an earlier investigation on the same preparation in which three different voltage-gated inward currents were found (Rivet et al., 1992). In particular, we confirm the presence of a further rapid calcium current (third-type), activated at more positive potentials than the T-type current. This current has so far only been found in cultured human skeletal myocytes (Rivet et al., 1992). Its average density was markedly increased in the HypoPP myotubes. Because of its presence also in normal myotubes this current component is unlikely to be caused by mutated L-type channels. We could not find a positive correlation between low L-type current amplitude and high third-type current amplitude in normal myotubes. This rules out the possibility that a cellular compensation mechanism generally leads to a strong third-type current whenever the L-type current is low. Yet, the mutation could alter calcium channel expression, e.g., delay downregulation of the third-type channel gene.

The significantly reduced amplitude of the L-type current density may most easily be explained by an elimination of the channel function by the point mutation. This may not be too surprising because the mutation is located in a domain which seems to be extremely important with regard to the modulation by calcium channel antagonistic drugs (see Catterall and Striessnig, 1992; Striessnig, Murphy, and Catterall, 1991). However, if both the normal and the mutant gene were producing α_1-proteins (normal and nonfunctional) at the same expression rate, a reduction of the current density to no more than 50% should be expected.

A reduction to a considerably lower value might indicate an inhibitory effect of mutant channels on normal channels which could take place if the DHP receptor molecules were arranged in an oligomeric structure. Such an oligomeric arrangement might be the t-tubular tetrads (Block, Imagawa, Campbell, and Franzini-Armstrong, 1988) which are thought to consist of four DHP receptors interacting with one calcium release channel (ryanodine receptor).

If one modified monomer is sufficient to inhibit the function of the tetramer, which would be compatible with the dominant mode of inheritance of the disease (compare Steinmeyer, Lorenz, Pusch, Koch, and Jentsch, 1994), we would expect a current reduction to 6% of the normal value corresponding to the expected percentage of normally structured tetramers. However, the current was reduced to one third of the control value; this percentage could be explained by two modified monomers needed to destroy the function of the tetramer. Thus, the data would be compatible with models in which an interaction within a tetrad of DHP receptors (Lamb, 1992; Ríos, Karhanek, Ma, and Gonzáles, 1993) may be necessary for gating the L-type calcium current.

Because of the proposed dual function of the DHP receptor as calcium channel and control device for calcium release, the altered voltage sensor may also affect control of calcium release from the sarcoplasmic reticulum. Alteration of this control mechanism could also be involved in the observed clinical symptoms, i.e., paralytic attacks or permanent muscle weakness. How a fall in extracellular potassium is able to induce or to aggravate the channel dysfunction causing episodes of paralysis (Rüdel et al., 1984), is still unclear. The open questions will be further clarified by studies on both calcium currents and calcium transients in myotubes of patients and on heterologous expression of the mutant channels, contained in cells which the other four subunits of the pentameric complex required for a functional protein.

Calcium release in skeletal muscle is not dependent on calcium influx as is the case in cardiac muscle. The role of the slow L-type calcium inward current for muscle contraction is therefore unknown. HypoPP is an important system for defining the function of this current and refining the model for excitation-contraction coupling.

Acknowledgements

We thank S. Schäfer and M. Rudolf for culturing the myotubes, U. Richter for technical assistance, S. Plate for secretarial assistance, and the families whose participation made this study possible.

Dr. I. Sipos was Visiting Scientist at the Department of Applied Physiology and supported by the European Community and the University of Ulm. Fellowships were given by the Deutsche Forschungsgemeinschaft (Karin Jurkat-Rott, Roland Heine). This work was supported by the Deutsche Forschungsgemeinschaft (to Frank Lehmann-Horn, Werner Melzer) the European Community (to Laszlo Kovacs, Werner Melzer, Istvan Sipos), and the Muscular Dystrophy Association (to Frank Lehmann-Horn).

References

Beam, K. G., C. M. Knudson, and J. A. Powell. 1986. A lethal mutation in mice eliminates the slow calcium current in skeletal muscle cells. *Nature.* 320:168–170.

Block, B. A., T. Imagawa, K. P. Campbell, and C. Franzini-Armstrong. 1988. Structural evidence for direct interaction between the molecular components of the transverse tubule/sarcoplasmic reticulum junction in skeletal muscle. *Journal of Cell Biology.* 107:2587–2600.

Brinkmeier, H., J. V. Mutz, M. J. Seewald, I. Melzner, and R. Rüdel. 1993. Specific modifications of the membrane fatty acid composition of human myotubes and their effects on the muscular sodium channels. *Biochimica et Biophysica Acta.* 1145:8–14.

Catterall, W. A. 1988. Structure and function of voltage-sensitive ion channels. *Science.* 242:50–61.

Catterall, W. A., and J. Striessnig. 1992. Receptor sites for Ca^{2+} channel antagonists. *Trends in Pharmacology Science.* 13:256–262.

Chaudhari, N. 1992. A single nucleotide in the skeletal muscle-specific calcium channel transcript of muscular dysgenesis (mdg) mice. *Journal of Biological Chemistry.* 267:25636–25639.

Drouet, B., L. Garcia, D. Simon-Chazottes, M. G. Mattei, J.-L. Guénet, A. Schwartz, G. Varadi, and M. Pinçon-Raymond. 1993. The gene encoding for the α_1 subunit of the skeletal dihydrophyridine receptor (Cchlla3 = mdg) maps to mouse chromosome 1 and human 1q32. *Mammalian Genome.* 4:499–503.

Fontaine, B., J. M. Vale Santos, K. Jurkat-Rott, J. Reboul, E. Plassart, C. S. Rime, A. Elbaz, R. Heine, J. Guimaraes, J. Weissenbach, N. Baumann, M. Fardeau, and F. Lehmann-Horn. 1994. Mapping of hypokalemic periodic paralysis (HypoPP) to chromosome 1q31-q32 by a genome-wide search in three European families. *Nature Genetics.* 6:267–272.

Gyapay, G., J. Morissette, A. Vignal, C. Dib, C. Fizames, P. Millasseau, S. Marc, G. Bernardi, M. Lathrop, and J. Weissenbach. 1994. The 1993-94 Généthon human genetic linkage map. *Nature Genetics.* 7:246–338.

Heine, R., U. Pika, and F. Lehmann-Horn. 1993. A novel SCN4A mutation causing myotonia aggravated by cold and potassium. *Human Molecular Genetics.* 2:1349–1353.

Hofmann, F., M. Biel, and V. Flockerzi. 1994. Molecular basis for Ca^{2+} channel diversity. *Annual Review of Neuroscience.* 17:399–418.

Hogan K., P. A. Powers, and R. G. Gregg. 1994. Cloning of human skeletal muscle $\alpha 1$ subunit of the dihydrophyridine-sensitive L-type calcium channel (CACNL1A3) *Genomics.* 24:608–609.

Jurkat-Rott, K., F. Lehmann-Horn, A. Elbaz, R. Heine, R. G. Gregg, K. Hogan, P. Powers, P. Lapie, J. E. Vale-Santos, J. Weissenbach, and B. Fontaine. 1994. A calcium channel mutation causing hypokalemic periodic paralysis. *Human Molecular Genetics.* 3:1415–1419.

Lamb, G. D. 1992. DHP receptors and excitation-contraction coupling. *Journal of Muscle Research and Cell Motility.* 13:394–405.

Lehmann-Horn, F., A. Engel, R. Rüdel, and K. Ricker. 1994. The periodic paralyses. *In* Myology. Second edition. A. G. Engel and C. Franzini-Armstrong, editors. McGraw-Hill, New York. 1304–1334.

Mori, Y., T. Niidome, Y. Fujita, M. Mynlieff, R. T. Dirksen, K. G. Beam, N. Iwabe, T. Miyata, D. Furutama, T. Furuichi, and K. Mikoshiba. 1993. Molecular diversity of voltage-dependent calcium channel. *Annals of the New York Academy of Sciences.* 707:87–108.

Ptácek, L., R. Tawil, R. C. Griggs, A. Engel, R. B. Layzer, H. Kwiencinski, P. G. McManis, L. Santiago, M. Moore, G. Fouad, P. Bradley, and M. F. Leppert. 1994. Dihydropyridine receptor mutations cause hypokalemic periodic paralysis. *Cell.* 77:863–868.

Ríos, E., M. Karhanek, J. Ma, and A. Gonzáles. 1993. An allosteric model of the molecular interactions of excitation-contraction coupling in skeletal muscle. *Journal of General Physiology.* 102:449–481.

Rivet, M., C. Cognard, N. Imbert, Y. Rideau, G. Duport, and G. Raymond. 1992. A third type of calcium current in cultured human skeletal muscle cells. *Neuroscience Letters.* 138:97–102.

Rüdel, R., F. Lehmann-Horn, K. Ricker, and G. Küther. 1994. Hypokalemic periodic paralysis: in vitro investigation of muscle fiber membrane parameters. *Muscle Nerve.* 7:110–120.

Sipos, I., G. Szücs, A. Struk, F. Lehmann-Horn, and W. Melzer. 1994. Modified Ca^{2+} current in skeletal muscle of patients with hypokalemic periodic paralysis. *Pflügers Archiv.* 426:R85. (Abstr.)

Steinmeyer, K., C. Lorenz, M. Pusch, M. C. Koch, and T. J. Jentsch. 1994. Multimeric structure of ClC-1 chloride channel revealed by mutations in dominant myotonia congenita (Thomsen). *EMBO Journal.* 13:737–743.

Striessnig, J., B. J. Murphy, and W. A. Catterall. 1991. Dihydropyridine receptor of L-type Ca^{2+} channels: identification of binding domains for [^{3}H] (+) -PN200-110 and [^{3}H] azidpoine within the α_1 subunit. *Proceedings of the National Academy of Sciences, USA.* 88:10769–10773.

Tanabe, T., H. Takeshima, A. Mikami, V. Flockerzi, H. Takahashi, K. Kangawa, M. Kojima, H. Matsuo, T. Hirose, and S. Numa. 1987. Primary structure of the receptor for calcium channel blockers from skeletal muscle. *Nature.* 328:313–318.

Tanabe, T., K. G. Beam, J. A. Powell, and S. Numa. 1988. Restoration of excitation-contraction coupling and slow calcium current in dysgenic muscle by dihydropyridine receptor complementary DNA. *Nature.* 336:134–139.

Tanabe, T., A. Mikami, T. Niidome, S. Numa, B. A. Adams, and K. G. Beam. 1993. Structure and function of voltage-dependent calcium channels from muscle. *Annals of the New York Academy of Sciences.* 707:81–86.

Muscular Dysgenesis The Role of Calcium Channels in Muscle Development

Nirupa Chaudhari

Department of Physiology, Colorado State University, Fort Collins, Colorado 80523

Calcium (Ca) channels, and the ion fluxes they generate, regulate a diversity of critical cellular functions. In mammalian striated muscle, L-type Ca channels are essential components of the chain of events known as excitation-contraction (e-c) coupling (reviewed, Bean, 1989; Catterall, 1991; Franzini-Armstrong and Jorgensen, 1994). Electrical excitation of the sarcolemma and transverse (t) tubules is transduced to the sarcoplasmic reticulum (SR) to release stored Ca^{2+}. In skeletal muscle, the voltage sensor for this transduction is the t-tubular dihydropyridine (DHP) receptor, which also functions as a DHP-sensitive (L-type) Ca channel (Rios and Brum, 1987; Tanabe, Beam, Powell, and Numa, 1988). Ca channels are composed of a principal pore-forming α_1 subunit and three to four additional subunits that may serve structural or regulatory functions (reviewed, Campbell, Leung, and Sharp, 1988; Isom, De Jongh, and Catterall, 1994).

There are recent indications that hypokalemic periodic paralysis, a human genetic disease causing episodes of muscular weakness, may be traceable to mutations in the α_1 subunit of the skeletal muscle-specific Ca channel (Jurkat-Rott, et al., 1994; Ptáček et al., 1994). An animal model that has proven invaluable for studying Ca channels in skeletal muscle is the muscular dysgenesis (*mdg*) mouse. The mutation arose spontaneously (Gluecksohn-Waelsch, 1963) and assorts as a single autosomal recessive gene (Pai, 1965). While heterozygotes appear normal, homozygous mutant mice possess skeletal muscle which is completely paralyzed, leading to perinatal death from respiratory failure. Although the sarcolemma retains the ability to generate normal action potentials (Powell and Fambrough, 1973) and the sarcoplasmic reticulum (SR) is capable of sequestering and releasing stored Ca^{2+} (Bowden-Essein, 1972; Klaus, Scordilis, Rapalus, Briggs, and Powell, 1983), functional linkage between the two membrane systems is lacking. That is, paralysis of dysgenic skeletal muscle is attributed to a breakdown in e-c coupling (Klaus et al., 1983). In dysgenic muscle, there is a severe depletion of DHP binding sites (Pinçon-Raymond, Rieger, Fosset, and Lazdunski, 1985) and the DHP-sensitive L-type Ca^{2+} current is missing (Beam, Knudson, and Powell, 1986).

The first molecular level clue regarding the genetic defect in muscular dysgenesis came when Tanabe et al. (1988) showed that Restriction Fragment Length Polymorphisms (RFLPs) in the gene for the α_1 subunit of the DHP receptor associate with the mutant allele. Furthermore, experimental introduction of cDNA encoding the α_1 subunit into dysgenic myotubes led to the rescue of e-c coupling as well as to restoration of Ca^{2+} current (Tanabe et al., 1988). This finding was instrumental in establishing the common genetic origin of the voltage sensor for e-c coupling and the L-type Ca channel.

E-c Coupling Components in Muscular Dysgenesis: Biochemical Studies

E-c coupling in normal skeletal muscle occurs at triad junctions, sites where t tubule and sarcoplasmic reticulum (SR) membranes and their protein constituents are intimately juxtaposed. Using Western blots, Knudson, Chaudhari, Sharp, Powell, Beam, and Campbell, (1989) demonstrated that many key triadic proteins are present in dysgenic muscle. The SR proteins, calsequestrin, calcium release channel (ryanodine receptor) and the Ca^{2+}, Mg^{2+}-ATPase and were readily detected in dysgenic muscle membranes, although their concentrations were lower than in normal skeletal muscle. The α_2 subunit of the DHP receptor also was present, but the α_1 subunit could not be detected at all (Knudson et al., 1989).

In spite of the apparent lack of α_1 protein, a low concentration of 6.6 kb mRNA, hybridizing with skeletal α_1 cDNA, exists in dysgenic skeletal muscle (Chaudhari, 1992). DNA sequencing of partial cDNAs, corresponding to the dysgenic α_1 mRNA, demonstrated that a single basepair deletion exists within the fourth homology domain (Fig. 1, *asterisk*). Direct sequencing of PCR products was used to show that a

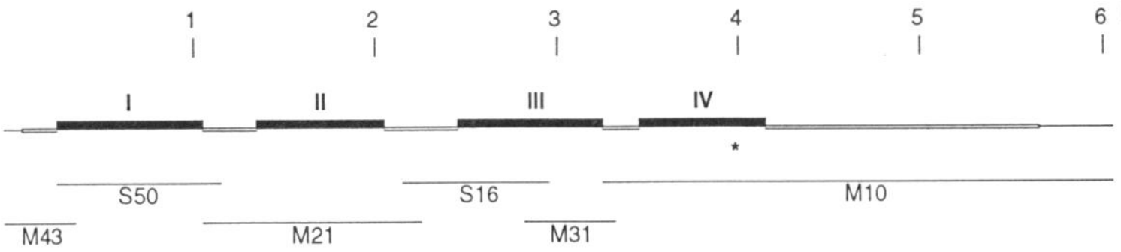

Figure 1. Schematic of cDNA clones encoding *mdg* skeletal calcium channel. (*Heavy line*) Full-length mRNA for the normal α_1 subunit, including the 5′ and 3′ untranslated regions (*single line*), the translated region (*double line*) and the four homologous repeats (*boxes I–IV*). cDNA clones isolated from libraries (*middle set of lines*) and by subcloning of PCR products (*bottom lines*) are shown. The asterisk denotes the site of the single base deletion. (*Hatch marks*) Denote length in kilobases above the mRNA. (Figure modified from Chaudhari, 1992.)

C residue is consistently deleted in α_1 mRNA from all affected (i.e., homozygous recessive) individuals (Chaudhari, 1992). The RFLPs in repeating domains I and III (Tanabe et al., 1988) do not map near the single-base deletion and presumably originated when the original mutation was bred into the present strain (129/ReJ) of mice.

The frame shift in the *mdg* skeletal α_1 mRNA occurs between the SS1 and SS2 segments of the fourth homology domain. These segments, located between the fifth and sixth transmembrane helices of each homology domain are thought to line the pore of voltage-gated cation channels (Guy and Conti, 1990). Important functional properties such as conductance, toxin block and ion selectivity can be altered by selected mutations in this region. The single-base deletion in *mdg* results in a shifted translational frame and premature termination. The resultant polypeptide is predicted to contain a stretch of 53 inappropriate amino acids beyond the deletion, with the concommitant loss of the SS2 and S6 segments of repeat IV as well as the entire cytoplasmic COOH terminus (Fig. 2).

Although the dysgenic α_1 mRNA is present at vanishingly low concentration in mutant muscle, higher molecular weight nuclear precursor RNAs are present at normal concentrations (Fig. 3 *A*) implying that the skeletal α_1 gene is transcribed at normal levels. The premature translational termination of the dysgenic α_1 mRNA leaves it with an excessively long 3′ untranslated tail that may make it subject to rapid degradation. Such mRNA instability after premature termination has also been noted for mutant mRNA in the muscular dystrophy (*mdx*) mouse (Sicinski, Geng, Ryder-Cook, Barnard, Darlison, and Barnard, 1989), and in a number of human genetic diseases (Dietz, Valle, Francomano, Kendzior, Pyeritz, and Cutting, 1993) and may proceed through a rapid 5′–3′ exonucleolytic pathway (Muhlrad and Parker, 1994).

The inability to detect a truncated α_1 polypeptide in dysgenic muscle by Western blots (Knudson et al., 1989) could reflect its very low concentration, owing to the low mRNA levels and/or to the degradation of a misfolded polypeptide. Alternatively, the antibodies used in the study (which were not epitope-mapped) might have recognized only the large cytoplasmic COOH terminus, which is missing in the *mdg* truncated polypeptide (Fig. 2).

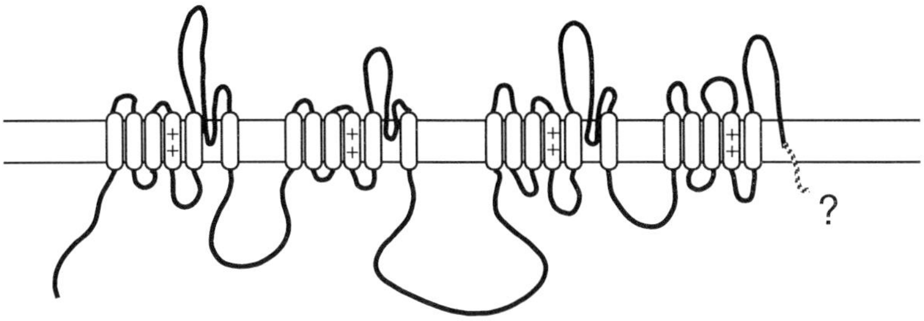

Figure 2. Hypothetical representation of the truncated *mdg* α_1 subunit predicted from cDNA clones. The typical pattern of four repeating homologous domains, each containing six transmembrane segments is shown. The fourth transmembrane helix in each repeat (S4) is marked + to indicate its probable role as voltage sensor. In *mdg,* the shifted reading frame after transmembrane segment 5 in repeat IV gives rise to a 53 amino acid tail (*hatched segment*) with no discernible similarity to sequences in voltage gated ion channels. The topology shown for this segment is strictly hypothetical and serves only to represent the possibility of an aberrantly folded α_1 subunit that could accumulate at low levels in *mdg* myotubes.

E-C Coupling in Muscular Dysgenesis: Electrophysiological Studies

Electrophysiological measurements of dysgenic myofibers demonstrated the loss of the typical skeletal L-type Ca^{2+} conductance (Beam et al., 1986). At the same time, dysgenic muscle cells possess a qualitatively distinct Ca^{2+} current, termed I_{dys} (Adams and Beam, 1989; Bournaud, Shimahara, Garcia, and Rieger, 1989). In myofibers from dysgenic animals, the mutant truncated α_1 polypeptide (Fig. 3) probably exists only at very low concentration and thus probably does not assemble into functional channels that might give rise to I_{dys}. Instead, it seems most likely that I_{dys} is generated by cardiac L-type channels because I_{dys} resembles the cardiac L-type current in characteristics such as activation kinetics, sensitivity to agonist and antagonist dihydropyridines and relative permeabilities to Ba^{2+} versus Ca^{2+} (Adams and Beam, 1989). Furthermore, this current, when pharmacologically potentiated, can support cardiac-type e-c coupling in dysgenic myotubes (Adams and Beam, 1991). The mRNA for the cardiac α_1 subunit is known to be expressed transiently in fetal skeletal muscle (Chaudhari and Beam, 1993) and is found at low concentration in skeletal myotubes for several days in culture (Yang and Chaudhari, 1993).

E-C Coupling Components in Muscular Dysgenesis: Morphological Studies

T tubules are invaginations of the surface membrane of mature skeletal myofibers. Triad junctions, the site of e-c coupling, are close appositions of t-tubular and SR

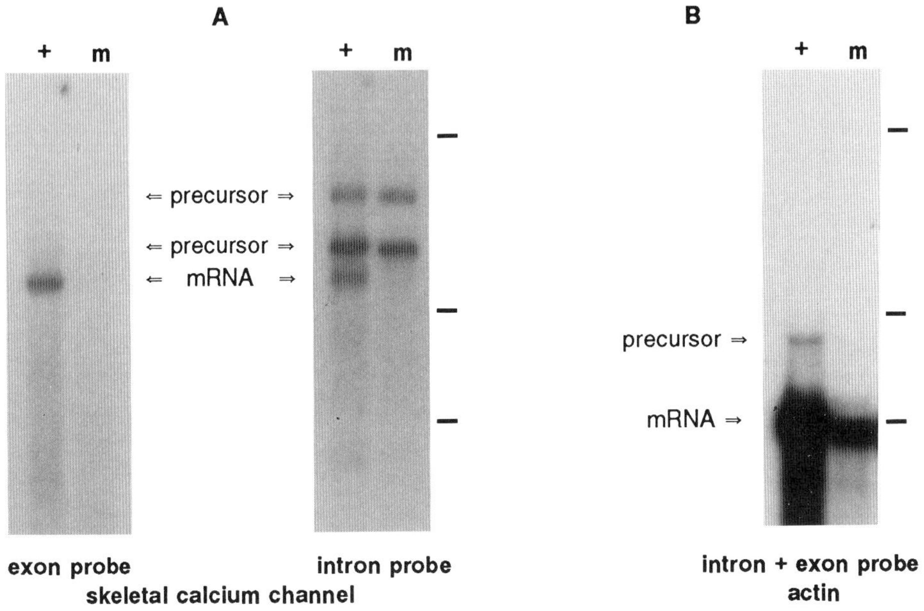

Figure 3. mRNA for skeletal α_1 is unstable although the gene is transcribed normally; other muscle-specific genes are transcribed at low levels. (*A*) Northern blot analysis of poly(*A*)RNA from normal (+) and dysgenic (*m*) neonatal skeletal muscle, hybridized with ^{32}P-labeled exonic or intronic probes. The mature mRNA of 6.6 kb is found at extremely low concentration in dysgenic muscle although the precursor RNAs, at 7.6 and 10.0 kb are present at normal levels. (*Hatch marks*) The positions of 45S (13.7 kb), 28S (5.1 kb) and 18S (1.9 kb) ribosomal RNAs as markers. (*B*) The same Northern blot was stripped and reprobed with a ^{32}P-labeled probe from the mouse skeletal α-actin gene ($\approx$60 bp of exon 1 and $\approx$580 bp of intron 1; Hu et al., 1986). Both the mature mRNA (1.7 kb) and a precursor RNA (3.4 kb) are present at lower concentration in dysgenic muscle relative to normal muscle of the same age. [Part *A* of figure from Chaudhari, 1992.]

membranes. The skeletal Ca channel of the t-tubular membrane and the ryanodine receptor of the SR, along with one or more additional proteins are concentrated in triads, as functional and/or structural components of the e-c coupling apparatus (reviewed, Franzini-Armstrong and Jorgensen, 1994). In spite of the persistence of many proteins involved in e-c coupling, t tubules and triads are rare in *mdg* myofibers (Pincon-Raymond et al., 1985; Franzini-Armstrong, Pincon-Raymond, and Rieger, 1991), implying that the α_1 polypeptide may play an obligatory role in the establishment of these membrane structures. On the other hand, Flucher, Andrews, Fleischer,

Marks, Caswell, and Powell (1993) and Flucher, Phillips, Powell, Andrews, and Daniels (1992) reported that in primary cultures of dysgenic myotubes, short patches of t tubules and triads do form after 2–3 wk of culture, implying that the skeletal Ca channel may not be an essential component of triads.

Curiously, the specific degradation (discussed above) of the α_1 mRNA does not occur in primary cultures established from dysgenic skeletal myoblasts. The mutant α_1 mRNA can be detected at near-normal concentration in cultured dysgenic myotubes (Chaudhari, unpublished observations) even though the paralytic phenotype is fully expressed in culture as in vivo (Beam et al., 1986). Thus, the truncated dysgenic α_1 polypeptide (Fig. 2) may be present at only limiting concentration in dysgenic myofibers in vivo, but may accumulate to significant levels in cultured dysgenic myotubes. Clearly, the truncated α_1 polypeptide is unable to carry out e-c coupling and ion permeation functions. However, it may be capable of structural and developmental roles (for instance in t-tubular and triad formation) as has been shown recently for an experimentally abbreviated α_1 polypeptide (Seigneurin-Venin, Song, Pincon-Raymond, Rieger, and Garcia, 1994). This may explain why secondary developmental effects such as the establishment of sarcomeric organization (Flucher et al., 1992) and the formation of t tubules and triads (compare Franzini-Armstrong et al., 1991; Flucher et al., 1993) in dysgenic myotubes progress farther in tissue culture than in vivo, especially after prolonged culturing. Franzini-Armstrong et al. (1991) had earlier postulated that residual amounts of Ca channel protein, if present in dysgenic muscle, might account for the sporadic triads detected.

Secondary Developmental Effects in Muscular Dysgenesis

Before the molecular definition of *mdg,* there was long-standing controversy over which aspects of the dysgenic phenotype were direct consequences of the mutation and which might be secondary effects. For instance, some authors had viewed the *mdg* mutation as primarily affecting neurons or neuromuscular components, based on the functional rescue of dysgenic myotubes upon coculture with normal spinal neurons (Rieger, Powell, and Pincon-Raymond, 1984; Rieger, Bournaud, Shimahara, Garcia, Pincon-Raymond, and Lazdunski, 1987; Pincon-Raymond, Murawsky, Mege, and Rieger, 1987). This interpretation was abandoned after the demonstration that normal fibroblasts fuse with dysgenic myotubes in culture, and that muscle-specific genes are then activated in the erstwhile fibroblast nuclei (Chaudhari, Delay, and Beam, 1989). The functional rescue of dysgenic myotubes during coculture with dissociated spinal cord cells probably reflected fusion with normal fibroblasts (an unavoidable contaminant in dissociated spinal cord) rather than a specific neuromuscular interaction.

The specific and primary loss of skeletal-specific Ca channels in *mdg* profoundly alters skeletal muscle, probably by altering developmental sequences of events and interactions. Some of the defects seen in dysgenic muscle may follow nonspecifically from muscle paralysis (i.e., may resemble effects of paralysis stemming from other causes). Defects in this category might include the immature morphology and multiple sites of motor nerve terminals on dysgenic fibers (Rieger and Pinçon-Raymond, 1981), the paucity of the high molecular weight form of acetyl cholinesterase in muscle (Rieger et al., 1984) and interruption of the normal program of motor neuron death (Oppenheim, Houenou, Pincon-Raymond, Powell, Rieger, and

Standish, 1986). These characteristics must be viewed as very indirectly ensuing from the primary loss of Ca channels.

Profound alterations in gene expression occur in *mdg* as a secondary consequence of the loss of Ca channels (Chaudhari and Beam, 1989). Normal skeletal muscle developing in vivo transcriptionally activates genes for muscle-specific contractile proteins, enzymes, pumps and ion channels around fetal day 12 in the mouse limb. After the onset of spontaneous twitch activity (fetal day 15), there is a pronounced increase in the mRNA levels (reflecting transcriptional activation) for this entire coordinately regulated set of genes. *Mdg* skeletal muscle, on the other hand, does not accumulate these same mRNAs above the pretwitch levels (Fig. 4 and Chaudhari and Beam, 1989). In *mdg* muscle, nuclear RNA precursors as well as mRNAs for such genes as α-actin are found at low concentration (Fig. 3 *B*), implying

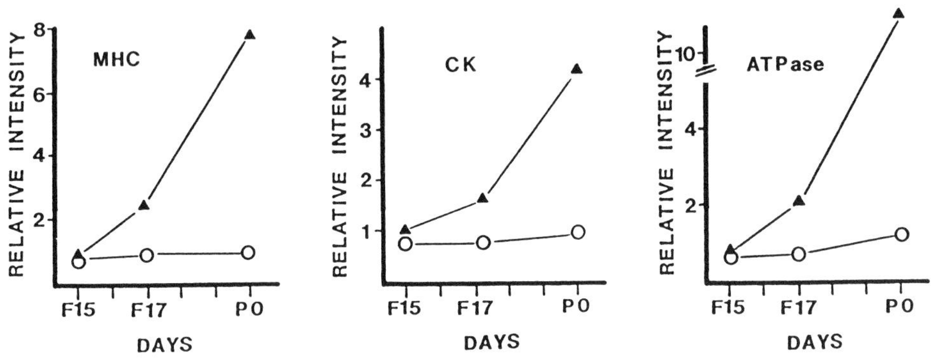

Figure 4. mRNAs for muscle-specific genes are upregulated after the onset of twitch in normal but not in dysgenic skeletal muscle. Northern blots, loaded with muscle poly(A)RNA from normal and dysgenic mice at the indicated fetal (*F*) and postnatal (*P*) days of development, were probed with ^{32}P-labeled probes for skeletal muscle-specific genes. mRNAs detected include a contractile protein, myosin heavy chain (MHC), muscle creatine kinase (CK) and the Ca^{2+} pump of SR (ATPase). Intensities of hybridizing bands, indicating mRNA concentration, were quantified by densitometry and demonstrate the consistent upregulation for all these mRNAs in normal muscle, after the initiation of twitch in vivo at fetal day 15. mRNA concentrations in dysgenic muscle remain at pretwitch levels. (Figure adapted from Chaudhari and Beam, 1989.)

that mRNA levels are low because of low transcriptional levels. This is in marked contrast to the normal transcription followed by mRNA instability in the case of the Ca channel α_1 subunit (Fig. 3 *A*). Transcriptional regulation of nicotinic acetylcholine receptors in muscle by electrical activity is known to involve surface Ca channels (Walke, Staple, Adams, Gnegy, Chahine, and Goldman, 1994; Huang, Flucher, Schmidt, Stroud, and Schmidt, 1994). Although such depolarization-transcription coupling has not directly been demonstrated for the larger set of muscle-specific genes, the pattern of gene expression in *mdg* would support such a model. This would be in keeping with the known regulation of differentiation by Ca channel activity in a number of other excitable cell types (reviewed, Spitzer, Gu, and Olson, 1994).

In terms of the gross pattern of gene expression, *mdg* muscle may be viewed as arrested at a fetal stage of development (Chaudhari and Beam, 1989). It is possible that some of the light and electron microscopically visible defects of dysgenic muscle, including the loss of sarcomeric organization (Pai, 1965; Platzer and Glueckson-Waelsh, 1972), may in part be attributable to the low concentrations of the gene products that are necessary for establishing the specialized filamentous and membrane structures of muscle.

The elucidation of the molecular basis for the muscular dysgenesis mutation has clarified our understanding of the mutant phenotype. The various phenotypic characteristics of mutant muscle can now be interpreted more accurately. The dysgenic myotube, a powerful expression system for the heterologous expression of recombinant Ca channels (e.g., Tanabe et al., 1988, 1991) has been established as a true null background. Equally importantly, the pervasive role of Ca channels in the development of skeletal muscle can be dissected using this valuable model system.

Acknowledgments

Supported by National Institutes of Health grant GM42652.

References

Adams, B. A., and K. G. Beam. 1989. A novel calcium current in dysgenic skeletal muscle. *Journal of General Physiology.* 94:429–444.

Adams, B. A., and K. G. Beam. 1991. Contractions of dysgenic skeletal muscle triggered by a potentiated, endogenous calcium current. *Journal of General Physiology.* 97:687–696.

Beam, K. G., C. M. Knudson, and J. A. Powell. 1986. A lethal mutation in mice eliminates the slow calcium current in skeletal muscle cells. *Nature.* 320:168–170.

Bean, B. P. 1989. Classes of calcium channels in vertebrate cells. *Annual Review of Physiology.* 51:367–384.

Bournaud, R., T. Shimahara, L. Garcia, and F. Rieger. 1989. Appearance of the slow Ca conductance in myotubes from mutant mice with "muscular dysgenesis". *Pflügers Archiv.* 414:410–415.

Bowden-Essien, F. 1972. An in vitro study of normal and mutant myogenesis in the mouse. *Deveopmental Biology.* 27:351–364.

Campbell, K. P., A. T. Leung, and A. H. Sharp. 1988. The biochemistry and molecular biology of the dihydropyridine-sensitive calcium channel. *Trends in Neurosciences.* 11:425–430.

Catterall, W. A. 1991. Excitation-contraction coupling in vertebrate skeletal muscle: a tale of two calcium channels. *Cell.* 64:871–874.

Chaudhari, N. 1992. A single nucleotide deletion in the skeletal muscle-specific calcium channel transcript of muscular dysgenesis (*mdg*) mice. *Journal of Biological Chemistry.* 267: 25636–25639.

Chaudhari, N., and K. G. Beam. 1989. The muscular dysgenesis mutation in mice leads to arrest of the genetic program for muscle differentiation. *Developmental Biology.* 133:456–467.

Chaudhari, N., and K. G. Beam. 1993. mRNA for cardiac calcium channel is expressed during development of skeletal muscle. *Developmental Biology.* 155:507–515.

Chaudhari, N., R. Delay, and K. G. Beam. 1989. Restoration of normal function in genetically defective myotubes by spontaneous fusion with fibroblasts. *Nature.* 341:445–447.

Dietz, H. C., D. Valle, C. A. Francomano, R. J. Kendzior, R. E. Pyeritz, and G. R. Cutting.

1993. The skipping of constitutive exons in vivo induced by nonsense mutations. *Science.* 259:680–683.

Flucher, B. E., S. B. Andrews, S. Fleischer, A. R. Marks, A. Caswell, and J. A. Powell. 1993. Triad formation: organization and function of the sarcoplasmic reticulum calcium release channel and triadin in normal and dysgenic muscle in vitro. *Journal of Cell Biology.* 123:1161–1174.

Flucher, B. E., J. L. Phillips, J. A. Powell, S. B. Andrews, and M. P. Daniels. 1992. Coordinated development of myofibrils, sarcoplasmic reticulum and transverse tubules in normal and dysgenic mouse skeletal muscle, *in vivo* and *in vitro. Developmental Biology.* 150:266–280.

Franzini-Armstrong, C., and A. O. Jorgensen. 1994. Structure and development of E-C coupling units in skeletal muscle. *Annual Review of Physiology.* 56:509–534.

Franzini-Armstrong, C., M. Pincon-Raymond, and F. Rieger. 1991. Muscle fibers from dysgenic mouse *in vivo* lack a surface component of peripheral couplings. *Developmental Biology.* 146:364–376.

Gluecksohn-Waelsch, S. 1963. Lethal genes and analysis of differentiation. *Science.* 142:1269–1276.

Guy, H. R., and F. Conti. 1990. Pursuing the structure and function of voltage-gated channels. *Trends in Neurosciences.* 13:201–206.

Hu, M. C.-T., S. B. Sharp, and N. Davidson. 1986. The complete sequence of the mouse skeletal α-actin gene reveals several conserved and inverted repeat sequences outside of the protein-coding region. *Molecular and Cellular Biology.* 6:15–25.

Huang, C.-F., B. E. Flucher, M. M. Schmidt, S. K. Stroud, and J. Schmidt. 1994. Depolarization-transcription signals in skeletal muscle use calcium flux through L channels, but bypass the sarcoplasmic reticulum. *Neuron.* 13:167–177.

Isom, L. L., K. S. De Jongh, and W. A. Catterall. 1994. Auxiliary subunits of voltage-gated ion channels. *Neuron.* 12:1183–1194.

Jurkat-Rott, K., F. Lehmann-Horn, A. Elbaz, R. Heine, R. G. Gregg, K. Hogan, P. A. Powers, P. Lapie, J. E. Vale-Santos, J. Weissenbach, and B. Fontaine. 1994. A calcium channel mutation causing hypokalemic periodic paralysis. *Human Molecular Genetics.* 3:1415–1419.

Klaus, M. M., S. P. Scordilis, J. M. Rapalus, R. T. Briggs, and J. A. Powell. 1983. Evidence for dysfunction in the regulation of cytosolic Ca^{++} in excitation-contraction uncoupled dysgenic muscle. *Developmental Biology.* 99:152–165.

Knudson, C. M., N. Chaudhari, A. H. Sharp, J. A. Powell, K. G. Beam, and K. P. Campbell. 1989. Specific absence of the α_1 subunit of the dihydropyridine receptor in mice with muscular dysgenesis. *Journal of Biological Chemistry.* 264:1345–1348.

Muhlrad, D., and R. Parker. 1994. Premature translational termination triggers mRNA decapping. *Nature.* 370:578–581.

Oppenheim, R. W., L. Houenou, M. Pincon-Raymond, J. A. Powell, F. Rieger, and L. J. Standish. 1986. The development of motoneurons in the embryonic spinal cord of the mouse mutant, *muscular dysgenesis (mdg/mdg):* survival, morphology, and biochemical differentiation. *Developmental Biology.* 114:426–436.

Pai, A. C. 1965. Developmental genetics of a lethal mutation, muscular dysgenesis (*mdg*), in the mouse. 1. Genetic analysis and gross morphology. *Developmental Biology.* 11:82–92.

Pincon-Raymond, M., M. Murawsky, R.-M. Mege, and F. Rieger. 1987. Abnormal enwrapment of intramuscular axons by distal Schwann cells with defective basal lamina in the muscular dysgenic mouse embryo. *Developmental Biology*. 124:259–268.

Pincon-Raymond, M., F. Rieger, M. Fosset, and M. Lazdunski. 1985. Abnormal transverse tubule system and abnormal amount of receptors for Ca^{++} channel inhibitors of the dihydropyridine family in skeletal muscle from mice with embryonic muscular dysgenesis. *Developmental Biology*. 112:458–466.

Platzer, A. C., and S. Gluecksohn-Waelsch. 1972. Fine structure of mutant (muscular dysgenesis) embryonic mouse muscle. *Developmental Biology*. 28:242–252.

Powell, J. A., and D. M. Fambrough. 1973. Electrical properties of normal and dysgenic mouse skeletal muscle in culture. *Journal of Cell Physiology*. 82:21–38.

Ptáček, L. J., R. Tawil, R. C. Griggs, A. G. Engel, R. B. Layzer, H. Kwiecinski, P. G. McManis, L. Santiago, M. Moore, G. Fouad, P. Bradley, and M. F. Leppert. 1994. Dihydropyridine receptor mutations cause hypokalemic periodic paralysis. *Cell*. 77:1–20.

Rieger, F., R. Bournaud, T. Shimahara, L. Garcia, M. Pincon-Raymond, and M. Lazdunski. 1987. Restoration of dysgenic muscle contraction and calcium channel function by co-culture with normal spinal cord neurons. *Nature*. 330:563–566.

Rieger, F., and M. Pincon-Raymond. 1981. Muscle and nerve in muscular dysgenesis in the mouse at birth: sprouting and multiple innervation. *Developmental Biology*. 87:85–101.

Rieger, F., J. A. Powell, and M. Pincon-Raymond. 1984. Extensive nerve overgrowth and paucity of the tailed asymmetric form (16 S) of acetylcholinesterase in the developing skeletal neuromuscular system of the dysgenic (*mdg/mdg*) mouse. *Developmental Biology*. 101:181–191.

Rios, E., and G. Brum. 1987. Involvement of dihydropyridine receptors in excitation-contraction coupling in skeletal muscle. *Nature*. 325:717–720.

Seigneurin-Venin, S., M. Song, M. Pinçon-Raymond, F. Rieger, and L. Garcia. 1994. Restoration of normal ultrastructure after expression of the α_1 subunit of the L-type Ca^{2+} channel in dysgenic myotubes. *FEBS Letters*. 342:129–134.

Sicinski, P., Y. Geng, A. S. Ryder-Cook, E. A. Barnard, M. G. Darlison, and P. J. Barnard. 1989. The molecular basis of muscular dystrophy in the *mdx* mouse: a point mutation. *Science*. 244:1575–1580.

Spitzer, N. C., X. Gu, and E. Olson. 1994. Action potentials, calcium transients and the control of differentiation of excitable cells. *Current Opinion in Neurobiology*. 4:70–77.

Tanabe, T., K. G. Beam, J. A. Powell, and S. Numa. 1988. Restoration of excitation-contraction coupling and slow calcium current in dysgenic muscle by dihydropyridine receptor complementary DNA. *Nature*. 336:134–139.

Walke, W., J. Staple, L. Adams, M. Gnegy, K. Chahine, and D. Goldman. 1994. Calcium-dependent regulation of rat and chick muscle nicotinic acetylcholine receptor (nAChR) gene expression. *Journal of Biological Chemistry*. 269:19447–19456.

Yang, Y., and N. Chaudhari. 1993. Detection of the cardiac calcium channel mRNA in developing skeletal muscle by *in situ* hybridization. *Society for Neuroscience Abstracts*. 19:1331. (Abstr.)

Chapter 5

Anion Channel Diseases

Function and Dysfunction of the CFTR Chloride Channel

J. W. Hanrahan,* J. A. Tabcharani,* F. Becq,* C. J. Mathews* O. Augustinas,‡ T. J. Jensen,§ X.-B. Chang,§ and J. R. Riordan§

**Department of Physiology, McGill University, Montréal, Québec, Canada H3G 1Y6; ‡Research Institute, Hospital for Sick Children, Toronto, Ontario M5G 1X8; and §S. C. Johnson Medical Research Center, Mayo Clinic Scottsdale, Scottsdale, Arizona 85259*

Cystic fibrosis (CF) is a common fatal genetic disease characterized by defective chloride transport across epithelia of the airways, exocrine ducts and intestine (Quinton, 1990). The mutated gene that causes CF, which was identified by positional cloning in 1989 (Rommens et al., 1989), encodes a protein named cystic fibrosis transmembrane conductance regulator (CFTR; Riordan et al., 1989). Although the precise function of CFTR was not apparent initially, a new cAMP-stimulated Cl conductance appeared when its gene was heterologously expressed in nonepithelial cells (Anderson, Berger, Rich, Gregory, Smith, and Welsh, 1991; Kartner et al., 1991). Using recombinant baculovirus-infected Sf9 insect cells, this conductance was found to be mediated by a nonrectifying Cl channel having low conductance, distinctive slow kinetics, and weak sensitivity to DIDS. The channel was indistinguishable from those in the apical membrane of T_{84} cells (Tabcharani, Low, Elie, and Hanrahan, 1990), a chloride-secreting cell line, and on pancreatic duct (Gray et al., 1989) and thyroid epithelial cells (Champigny et al., 1990). The same channel also appeared when CFTR was expressed in CHO cells (Fig. 1; Tabcharani, Chang, Riordan, and Hanrahan, 1991) or *Xenopus* oocytes (Bear, Duguay, Naismith, Kartner, Hanrahan, and Riordan, 1991). Based on similarities at the single-channel level, including PKA regulation, unitary conductance, gating and pharmacology, CFTR was proposed to be the low-conductance Cl channel (Kartner et al., 1991).

Further evidence that CFTR mediates a Cl conductance came from whole-cell patch clamp studies. Anderson et al. (1991) found that mutations in the first and sixth predicted transmembrane segments altered the selectivity of whole-cell anion currents. Finally, when CFTR was purified to homogeneity from Sf9 insect cells and reconstituted into planar lipid bilayers, it formed low-conductance Cl channels like those on CFTR-expressing cells (Bear, Li, Kartner, Bridges, Jensen, Ramjeesingh, and Riordan, 1992). Although CFTR channels have been reported in cardiac and other cell types and may have other functions in addition to serving as a plasma membrane chloride channel, most disease symptoms can be explained as primary or secondary consequences of a deficiency in epithelial Cl conductance.

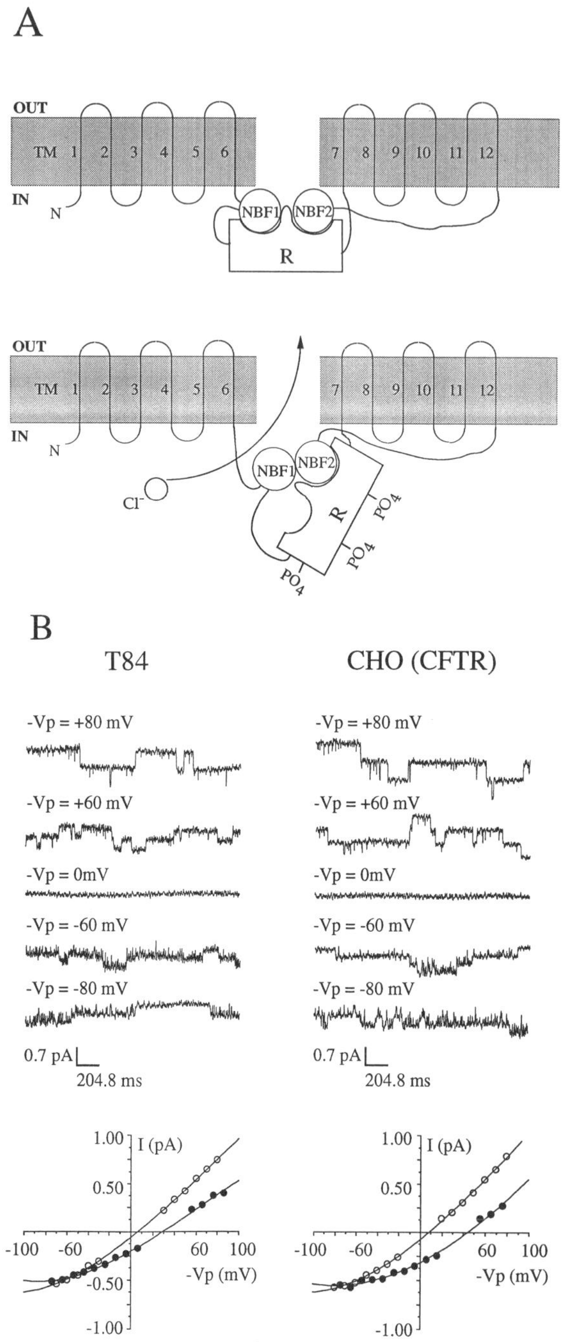

FIGURE 1. (*A*) Cartoon of CFTR showing major domains and speculations regarding the effect of phosphorylation. Note that inhibition by the regulatory (R) domain is relieved by phosphorylation while nucleotide binding folds (NBFs) are allowed to interact. (*B*) Comparison of single Cl channels activated by cAMP in T_{84} cells expressing endogenous CFTR, and in CHO cells after transfection with CFTR. Taken from Hanrahan et al. (1993).

Regulation of the CFTR Cl Channel by Phosphorylation

CFTR has 10 high affinity consensus sequences for cAMP-dependent protein kinase (PKA) defined as R/K,R/K,X,S/T, consistent with its role as a regulated Cl channel. Channel activity declines rapidly after patches are excised from cAMP stimulated CHO cells into solutions containing MgATP (Fig. 2; 37°C; Tabcharani et al., 1991). This does not occur in the presence of PKA and can be reversed by addition of this kinase. In contrast, addition of PKC and DiC_8 produce only small stimulations (to $P_o \approx 0.08$ vs 0.4), although they greatly increase the rate and magnitude of subsequent PKA responses. The R domain contains 9 of the 10 strict consensus sequences for PKA and 7 of the 29 predicted PKC sites on CFTR. Potentiation by

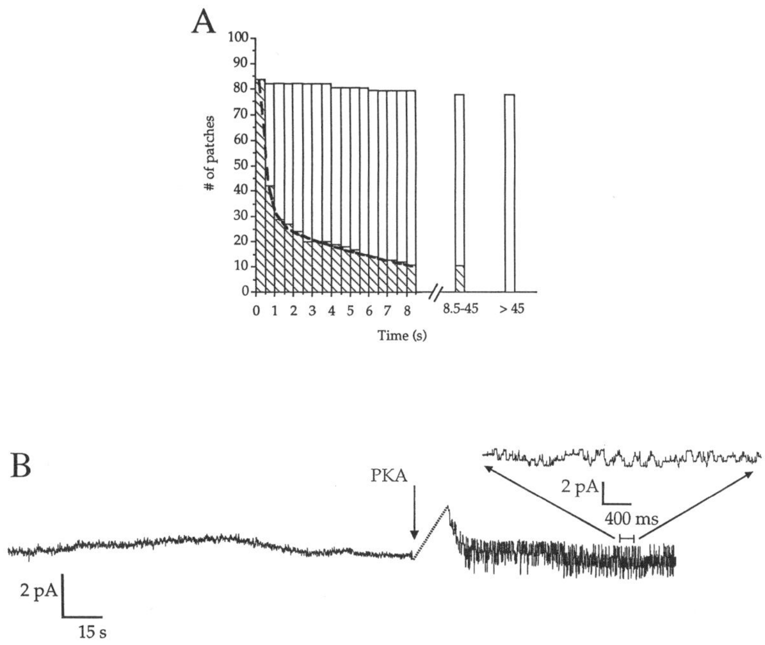

FIGURE 2. (*A*) Rundown of CFTR channel activity after excision from CHO cells in the presence of MgATP or MgATP + PKA at 37°C. Channel activity was assessed in 500 ms intervals in 84 patches excised in the presence (*open bars*) or absence (*hatched bars*) of PKA. (*B*) Restimulation of CFTR channels by PKA after rundown in excised patch. Taken from Tabcharani et al. (1991).

PKC may reflect a subtle conformational change in the R domain that causes more sites to be accessible to PKA. PKA-mediated phosphorylation does alter the secondary structure of recombinant R domain as measured by circular dicroism spectroscopy (Dulhanty and Riordan, 1994). PKC alone does not cause detectable alterations in structure, however, its effect on PKA-induced changes have not been studied.

Mutagenesis and patch clamp studies indicate that none of the strong PKA sites are essential for activation because a mutant lacking all 10 major consensus sequences (10SA) can still be phosphorylated and activated by PKA. Phosphorylation of 10SA is reduced by ~98% and P_o is reduced by ~75% compared to wild-type CFTR (Chang, Tabcharani, Hou, Jensen, Kartner, Alon, Hanrahan, and Riordan,

1993). The channel activity of phosphorylation site mutants is roughly proportional to the number of PKA sites remaining. This progressive phosphorylation at multiple sites may be a way of providing graded responses to hormonal stimuli. It has been proposed that the level of phosphorylation determines whether ATP hydrolysis is required to close the channel (Hwang, Horie, and Gadsby, 1993; Hwang, Baukrowitz, Nagel, Horie, and Gadsby, 1994).

PKA regulation is complex, with some sites having larger effects on P_o than others. At least one site (ser^{660}) may be inhibitory. Channel activity can be reduced further by altering other potential PKA sites such as ser^{753} (Siebert et al., 1995) but it has not yet been possible to abolish PKA activation completely. Interestingly, potentiation of the PKA response by PKC is still observed after all 10 strict PKA sites are mutated (10SA). Thus, "cryptic" PKA sites may mediate residual PKA activation and also interactions between PKA and PKC. While PKA clearly phosphorylates CFTR, halide efflux and patch clamp studies do not exclude the possibility that some PKA responsiveness is due to the phosphorylation of other proteins that regulate CFTR.

Epithelial Cl secretion is triggered by cAMP and apical Cl conductance is the rate-limiting step in this process (Frizzell, Field, and Schultz, 1979), thus, activation by PKA is the main stimulus for CFTR in vivo. Indirect evidence that other kinases may modulate CFTR activity comes from the fact that channels gradually become less responsive to PKA after patches are excised, consistent with dephosphorylation at permissive (non-PKA) sites. The alkaline phosphatase inhibitor bromotetramisole inhibits CFTR dephosphorylation in isolated membranes and leads to activation of channels in cell-attached patches, even though G551D is a disease-causing mutation that prevents stimulation by forskolin (Becq, Jensen, Chang, Savoia, Rommens, Tsui, Buchwald, Riordan, and Hanrahan, 1994). Because bromotetramisole does not directly stimulate channels in excised patches, its stimulatory effect in the cell-attached configuration is most easily explained by cumulative phosphorylation by other (non-PKA) kinases in the cytosol. Whether these unidentified kinases are also responsible for the constitutive phosphorylation of CFTR seen in unstimulated cells (Cheng, Gregory, Marshall, Paul, Souza, White, O'Riordan, and Smith, 1990) is unknown. Tyrosine phosphorylation may inhibit CFTR activity because the tyrosine kinase inhibitor genistein stimulates halide efflux from T_{84} cells (Illek, Fischer, Santos, Widdicombe, Machen, and Reenstra, 1994) and from CFTR-expressing CHO cells, but not from control cells (Fig. 3). According to iodide efflux assays, the genistein response is additive to forskolin stimulation and is sensitive to the tyrosine phosphatase inhibitor vanadate, however, more studies are needed to assess whether genistein decreases tyrosine phosphorylation or has some other, less-specific mode of action. Multifunctional calcium-calmodulin kinase (CaMKII) does not stimulate CFTR channels when added to excised patches (Berger, Travis, and Welsh, 1993), consistent with the insensitivity of whole-cell CFTR currents to intracellular calcium in many cell types (Cliff and Frizzell, 1990; Worrell and Frizzell, 1991; Wagner, Cozens, Shulman, Gruenert, Stryer, and Gardner, 1991).

Dephosphorylation plays a dynamic role in regulating CFTR but the major phosphatases remain to be identified. Okadaic acid and calyculin A, which inhibit type 1 and type 2A protein phosphatases, do not affect CFTR activity in patches excised from CHO (Tabcharani et al., 1991; Becq et al., 1994) or pancreatic duct cells (Becq, Fanjul, Merton, Figarella, Hollande, and Gola, 1993). Although inhibiting

PP1 and PP2A does not affect channel activity in these preparations, they are clearly present in isolated CHO membranes because spontaneous dephosphorylation of CFTR protein is partially inhibited by okadaic acid. In cardiac cells, okadaic acid inhibits ~25% of the down regulation when cAMP is washed out, with the remaining 75% being okadaic acid insensitive (Hwang et al., 1993).

Rundown and dephosphorylation are observed in the nominal absence of calcium or calmodulin, therefore, it is unlikely that protein phosphatase 2B normally regulates CFTR. Protein phosphatase 2C (PP2C) remains a good candidate although to date there has been no direct evidence supporting its role. Exogenous alkaline phosphatase reduces open probability by 90% when added to excised patches in the presence of PKA and MgATP, and similar results have been obtained using acid phosphatase (F. Becq and J. Hanrahan, unpublished observations). The finding that channel activity is increased by exposure to a specific antibody against alkaline phosphatase suggests that the endogenous phosphatase resembles alkaline phosphatase (Becq et al., 1993). The phosphatases controlling CFTR may be less active in some cell lines than others (Berger, Anderson, Gregory, Thompson, Howard,

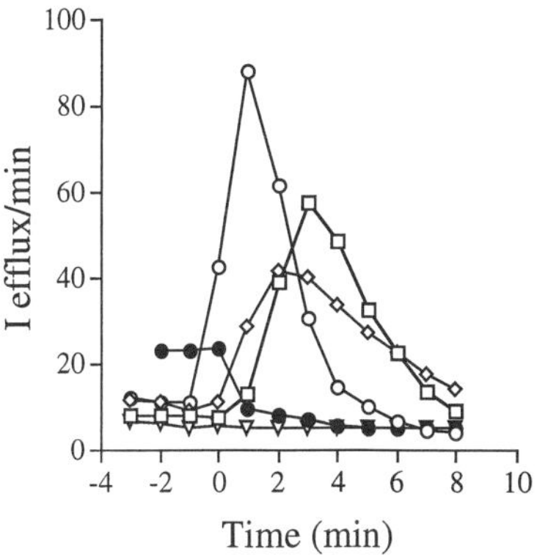

FIGURE 3. Effect of (□) forskolin, (◇) genistein, (○) forskolin + genistein, and (▽) genistein + vanadate on iodide efflux from transfected CHO cells. Forskolin + genistein did not stimulate efflux from control CHO cells lacking CFTR.

Maurer, Mulligan, Smith, and Welsh, 1991) and it will be interesting to determine whether cell-specific kinase or phosphatase activities contribute to the variable severity of CF symptoms among different tissues such as lung and heart, or the constitutively high activity of CFTR in sweat ducts (Quinton, 1983) and Calu-3 submucosal gland airway cells (Haws, Finkbeiner, Widdicombe, and Wine, 1993).

CFTR Gating Depends on ATP Hydrolysis

Phosphorylated CFTR channels need hydrolyzable nucleotides to become active (Fig. 4; see Anderson, Gregory, Thompson, Souza, Paul, Mulligan, Smith, and Welsh, 1991; Anderson and Welsh, 1992; Nagel et al., 1992). Quinton and Reddy (1992) found that CFTR-mediated Cl conductance in permeabilized sweat ducts can be elevated by poorly hydrolyzable ATP analogues such as AMP-PNP when low concentrations of ATP are also present. This has been explained at the single-channel level by the finding that CFTR channels enter a prolonged open burst state in mixtures of ATP and nucleotide analogues (Fig. 4; see Hwang et al., 1994; Gunderson and Kopito, 1994) or pyrophosphate (Baukrowitz, Hwang, Nairn, and

Gadsby, 1994; Gunderson and Kopito, 1994). Similar results are obtained when channels are exposed to orthovanadate or berylium fluoride (Baukrowitz et al., 1994), which inhibit ATPases by binding tightly in place of inorganic phosphate (P_i) after cleavage of the γ-phosphate bond. The relationship between ATP concentration and open probability suggests that ATP binds to CFTR at two or more sites, and that association at one site may inhibit binding at the other (Anderson and Welsh, 1992; Gunderson and Kopito, 1994). Fluorescence, patch clamp, and microelectrode studies of channels bearing mutations that should inhibit ATP binding or hydrolysis indicate that the functions of nucleotide binding folds are not equivalent (Anderson and Welsh, 1992; Smit, Wilkinson, Mansoura, Collins, and Dawson, 1993) and that hydrolysis at NBF2 is not required for the channel to open (Gregory, Rich, Cheng, Souza, Paul, Manavalan, Anderson, Welsh, and Smith, 1991).

A reaction scheme has been proposed to explain the gating of CFTR channels in heart cells (Baukrowitz et al., 1994; Hwang et al., 1994). According to this model, hydrolysis at one site (NBD-A) opens the channel, which then remains in an open

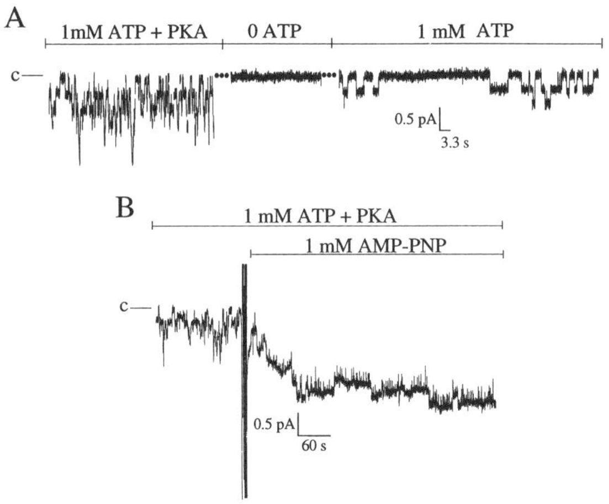

FIGURE 4. (*A*) Restimulation of CFTR channel activity by ATP alone after phosphorylation by PKA + MgATP. Traces are interrupted during solution changes. (*B*) Prolonged open burst state induced by addition of AMP-PNP in the presence of ATP.

burst state until ADP and Pi dissociate from NBD-A. When the channel is highly phosphorylated and open probability is high, channel closing becomes dependent on ATP hydrolysis at the second site (NBD-B), which enhances the release of hydrolysis products that were bound at NBD-A (Hwang et al., 1994). Thus, opening and closing transitions of CFTR channels are both coupled to ATP hydrolysis cycles, with the latter being dependent on interactions between nucleotide binding folds. The model can explain many observations and provides a useful framework for designing further experiments. Kinetic schemes comprised of two closed and one open state have been proposed for ATP regulated gating of phosphorylated channels (Winter, Sheppard, Carson, and Welsh, 1994; Gunderson and Kopito, 1994). The mechanism by which ATP hydrolysis leads to opening of the pore, and how disease mutations alter coupling between hydrolysis and gating remain exciting questions for the future.

Permeation in the CFTR Pore

The current-voltage relationship of single CFTR channels, which normally displays Goldman-type rectification on cell, became linear over the range ± 100 mV with conductance of 6.9 pS in excised patches bathed with symmetrical 154 mEq/liter chloride solutions (Hanrahan, Tabcharani, and Grygorczyk, 1993). The conductance of single channels is 8.7–9.6 pS at 37°C, 7.5–8.4 pS at 27°C, and 6.8–7.6 pS at room temperature. Polyatomic anions having diameters > 0.45 nm are impermeant, suggesting CFTR has a pore diameter of ~0.55 nm similar to ligand-gated (Bormann, Hamill, and Sakmann, 1987) and outwardly rectifying anion channels (Halm and Frizzell, 1992). ATP is reported to carry current through CFTR (Reisin, Prat, Abraham, Amara, Gregory, Ausiello, and Cantiello, 1994), although this has not been observed in all studies. When biionic reversal potentials are measured immediately after exposing the cytoplasmic side to test anions they yield the sequence $P_I(2.1) > P_{Br}(1.3) > P_{Cl}(1.0) > P_F(0.1)$, consistent with a "weak field strength" selectivity filter. However, iodide currents also become blocked within 1–2 min and the extrapolated reversal potential shifts strongly in the negative direction, indicating $P_I/P_{Cl} < 0.5$. Iodide block and hysteresis in the *I*/*V* relationship probably account for the low P_I/P_{Cl} permeability ratio measured macroscopically, which is used as a hallmark of CFTR conductance. The effects of iodide are not caused by trace I_3- or other polyiodides because they are still observed with iodide solutions containing 20 mM thiosulfate. Several lines of evidence indicate that TM1, TM5, TM6, and TM12 contribute to the pore region of CFTR (Anderson, Rich, Gregory, Smith, and Welsh, 1991; Akabas, Kaufmann, Cook, and Archdeacon, 1994; Mansoura, Strong, Collins, and Dawson, 1994; Tabcharani, Rommens, Hou, Chang, Tsui, Riordan, and Hanrahan, 1993; McDonough, Davidson, Lester, and McCarty, 1994). TM1 and TM6 peptides can form CFTR-like pores when reconstituted into planar bilayers (Oblatt-Montal, Reddy, Iwamoto, Tomich, and Montal, 1994). Overexpressing a construct comprising the first half of CFTR (i.e., the first six membrane-spanning regions, NBF1 and the R domain) generates Cl channels that have properties resembling wild-type CFTR (Sheppard, Ostegaard, Rich, and Welsh, 1994). Although permeation in the CFTR pore is still poorly understood, it is clear that permeation properties are altered by some disease-causing mutations (see below).

CF Mutations Can Be Grouped by Molecular Mechanism or by Phenotype

Fig. 5 shows examples of CFTR channels bearing the most common severe (F508Δ, G551D) and mild (R117H, R347H) CF mutations. Over 400 mutations have been identified in the CFTR gene, of which about three quarters probably cause CF (The CF Genetic Analysis Consortium, 1994). The molecular basis of CFTR dysfunction varies depending on the particular mutation (Tsui, 1992). Some CF mutations cause truncation or defective processing, whereas others cause CFTR to be unresponsive to PKA, or to have low open probability or reduced conductance (see **Smith, this volume**). Mutations may disrupt function at more than one level; for example, ΔF508 causes biosynthetic arrest (Cheng et al., 1990) and a reduced P_o (Dalemans, Barbry, Champigny, Jallat, Dott, Dreyer, Crystal, Pavirani, Lecocq, and Lazdunski, 1991). The severe mutation G551D does not block CFTR targeting or alter single-channel conductance, but channels with this mutation are less responsive to PKA, particularly in cell-attached patches.

Mutations can be classified according to the phenotype they produce. Approximately 15% of CF patients have relatively mild disease as defined by their level of pancreatic function (Kristidis, Bozen, Corey, Markiewicz, Rommens, Tsui, and Durie, 1992). These mild mutations include Y109C (Schaedel, Kristoffersson, Kornfält, and Holmberg, 1994), R117H, R334W, R347P, A455E, and P574H (see Tsui, 1992). Individuals with one chromosome bearing a mild mutation and the other a severe mutation display the mild phenotype (Rommens et al., 1989). Only a small number of mild mutations have been identified and they occur at low frequencies, but mild mutations are less likely to be diagnosed, therefore their incidence in the general population may be underestimated due to sampling bias.

R117H, which is in the first extracellular loop between TM1 and TM2, reduces open probability but has little, if any, effect on single-channel conductance at negative membrane potentials. It is intriguing that a mutation at this extracellular loop has such marked effects on the closing rate, when gating is normally controlled by phosphorylation and nucleotide interactions actions at the cytoplasmic side. It

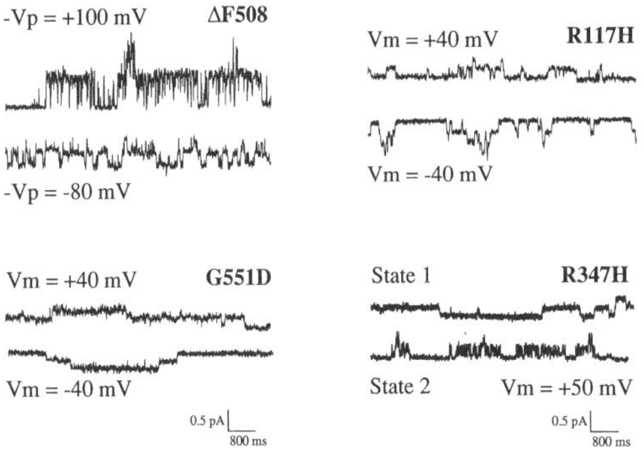

FIGURE 5. Recordings of mutant CFTR channels bearing the most common disease-causing mutations. Patients having R117H or R347H alleles have pancreatic sufficiency and relatively mild symptoms, ΔF508 and G551D are associated with a severe cystic fibrosis phenotype.

would not be surprising if Y109C, another mild mutation in this region, has similar effects on open probability. CF mutations in TM6 reduce single-channel conductance (Sheppard et al., 1993; Tabcharani et al., 1993) but may also reduce open probability as reported recently for G314E in TM5 (Mansoura et al., 1994). Many mutations in the NBFs cause severe CF by biosynthetic arrest and mislocalization of CFTR protein (Cheng et al., 1990). This also appears to be true for some mild mutations in NBF1 (e.g., A455E and P574H); these mutations generate little mature CFTR protein, but those channels that are produced have normal conductance and open probability (Ostedgaard et al., 1994).

The functional consequences of some mutations have been studied using excised, inside-out patches (Tabcharani et al., 1993). In wild-type CFTR channels, thiocyanate (SCN) causes fast, voltage-dependent block, consistent with an anion binding site ~19% of the way through the membrane field from the cytoplasmic side. This electrical distance coincides with the position of arg^{347} near the cytoplasmic end of the sixth predicted membrane-spanning helix. Mutating arg^{347} to aspartate (R347D) reduces single-channel conductance by 60% and abolishes voltage-dependent SCN block but does not induce significant outward rectification in the current-voltage

(I/V) curve. The surprising linearity of the I/V relationship suggests that the low conductance of R347D is not due to addition of a new barrier to anion flow (i.e., asp^-), but more likely reflects some fundamental change in the mechanism of permeation. To examine the possibility that occupancy is altered by the mutation, the conductance of R347D channels was measured in symmetrical solutions containing chloride and thiocyanate ($P_{SCN}/P_{Cl} = 1.5$). Raising the SCN mole fraction reduces, and then increases, the conductance of wild-type CFTR channels (Fig. 6). This "anomalous mole fraction effect," which provides evidence that the pore can contain more than one anion simultaneously, is abolished by substitutions that eliminate the positive charge at residue 347. Moreover, when this arginine is mutated to a histidine (R347H), multi-ion pore behavior can be toggled on and off by varying the pH. Thus, naturally occurring mutations at this residue in TM6, (which all lead to loss of

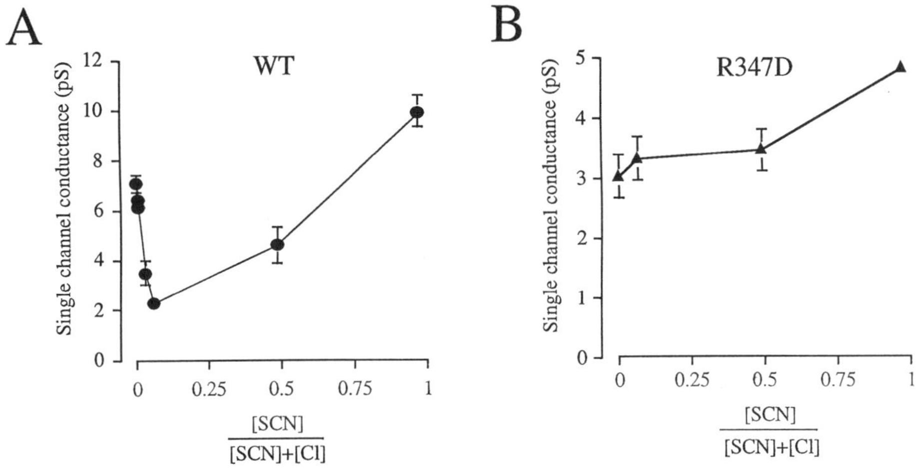

FIGURE 6. Evidence for the loss of multi-ion pore behavior induced by alterations at R347, a site of several known CF mutations. (*a*) Anomalous mole fraction effect in mixtures of chloride and thiocyanate; conductance is reduced and then increased by exposure to symmetrical solutions containing mixtures of SCN and Cl. (*b*) Monotonic increase in single-channel conductance of the R347D mutant when the SCN mole fraction is increased. Taken from Tabcharani et al. (1993).

positive charge; R347H, R347P, R347L), may cause cystic fibrosis in part by reducing channel occupancy, i.e., by converting CFTR from a multi-ion to a single-ion pore (Tabcharani et al., 1993).

Conclusions

The combination of mutagenesis and electrophysiological analysis should continue providing new insights into structure/function relations of the CFTR pore and should also help test the models that have been proposed recently for CFTR gating. The precise role of each NBF remains uncertain, and studies of interactions between domains, such as transduction of ATP hydrolysis energy to the channel gate, are just beginning. The transmembrane segments and loops that comprise the pore need to be characterized more fully. Because alterations at critical locations are likely to cause malfunction and cystic fibrosis, examining the consequences of disease-associated mutations may be a useful approach for locating regions of the protein that are important for anion permeation and at particular steps in the reaction scheme.

References

Akabas, M. H., C. Kaufmann, T. A. Cook, and P. Archdeacon. 1994. Amino acid residues lining the chloride channel of the cystic fibrosis transmembrane conductance regulator. *Journal of Biological Chemistry*. 269:14865–14868.

Anderson, M. P., H. A. Berger, D. P. Rich, R. J. Gregory, A. E. Smith, and M. J. Welsh. 1991. Nucleoside triphosphates are required to open the CFTR chloride channel. *Cell.* 67:775–784.

Anderson, M. P., R. J. Gregory, S. Thompson, D. W. Souza, S. Paul, R. C. Mulligan, A. E. Smith, and M. J. Welsh. 1991. Demonstration that CFTR is a chloride channel by alteration of its anion selectivity. *Science*. 253:202–205.

Anderson, M. P., D. P. Rich, R. J. Gregory, A. E. Smith, and M. J. Welsh. 1991. Generation of cAMP-activated chloride currents by expression of CFTR. *Science*. 251:679–682.

Anderson, M. P., and M. J. Welsh. 1992. Regulation by ATP and ADP of CFTR chloride channels that contain mutant nucleotide-binding domains. *Science*. 257:1701–1704.

Baukrowitz, T., T.-C. Hwang, A. C. Nairn, and D. C. Gadsby. 1994. Coupling of CFTR Cl-channel gating to an ATP hydrolysis cycle. *Neuron*. 12:473–482.

Bear, C. E., F. Duguay, A. L. Naismith, N. Kartner, J. W. Hanrahan, and J. R. Riordan. 1991. Cl^- channel activity in *Xenopus* oocytes expressing the cystic fibrosis gene. *Journal of Biological Chemistry*. 266:19142–19145.

Bear, C. E., C. Li, N. Kartner, R. J. Bridges, T. J. Jensen, M. Ramjeesingh, and J. R. Riordan. 1992. Purification and functional reconstitution of the cystic fibrosis transmembrane conductance regulator (CFTR). *Cell.* 68:809–818.

Becq, F., M. Fanjul, M. Merten, C. Figarella, E. Hollande, and M. Gola. 1993. Possible regulation of CFTR chloride channels by membrane bound phosphatases in pancreatic duct cells. *FEBS Letters*. 327:337–342.

Becq, F., T. J. Jensen, X.-B. Chang, A. Savoia, J. M. Rommens, L.-C. Tsui, M. Buchwald, J. R. Riordan, and J. W. Hanrahan. 1994. Phosphatase inhibitors activate normal and defective CFTR chloride channels. *Proceedings of the National Academy of Sciences, USA*. 91:9160–9164.

Berger, H. A., M. P. Anderson, R. J. Gregory, S. Thompson, P. W. Howard, R. A. Maurer, R. Mulligan, A. E. Smith, and M. J. Welsh. 1991. Identification and regulation of the cystic fibrosis transmembrane conductance regulator-generated chloride channel. *Journal of Clinical Investigation*. 88:1422–1431.

Berger, H. A., S. M. Travis, and M. J. Welsh. 1993. Regulation of the cystic fibrosis transmembrane conductance regulator Cl^- channel by specific protein kinases and phosphatases. *Journal of Biological Chemistry*. 268:2037–2047.

Bormann, J., O. P Hamill, and B. Sakmann. 1987. Mechanism of anion permeation through channels gated by glycine and gamma-aminobutyric acid in mouse cultured spinal neurones. *Journal of Physiology*. 385:243–286.

Champigny, G., B. Verrier, C. Gérard, J. Mauchamp, and M. Lazdunski. 1990. Small conductance chloride channels in the apical membrane of thyroid cells. *FEBS Letters.* 259:263–268.

Chang, X.-B., J. A. Tabcharani, Y.-X. Hou, T. J. Jensen, N. Kartner, N. Alon, J. W. Hanrahan, and J. R. Riordan. 1993. Protein kinase A (PKA) still activates CFTR chloride channel after mutagenesis of all ten PKA consensus phosphorylation sites. *Journal of Biological Chemistry.* 268:11304–11311.

Cheng, S. H., R. J. Gregory, J. Marshall, S. Paul, D. W. Souza, G. A. White, C. R. O'Riordan, and A. E. Smith. 1990. Defective intracellular transport and processing of CFTR is the molecular basis of most cystic fibrosis. *Cell.* 63:827–834.

Cliff, W.H., and R.A. Frizzell. 1990. Separate Cl^- conductances activated by cAMP and Ca^{2+} in Cl^- secreting epithelial cells. *Proceedings of the National Academy of Sciences, USA.* 87:4956–4960.

The Cystic Fibrosis Genetic Analysis Consortium. 1994. Population variation of common cystic fibrosis mutations. Human Mutation. 4:167–177.

Dalemans, W., P. Barbry, G. Champigny, S. Jallat, K. Dott, D. Dreyer, R. G. Crystal, A. Pavirani, J.-P. Lecocq, and M. Lazdunski. 1991. Altered chloride ion channel kinetics associated with the deltaF508 cystic fibrosis mutation. *Nature.* 354:526–528.

Denning, G. M., M. P. Anderson, J. F. Amara, J. Marshall, A. E. Smith, and M. J. Welsh. 1992. Processing of mutant cystic fibrosis transmembrane conductance regulator is temperature-sensitive. *Nature.* 358:761–764.

Dulhanty, A. M. and J. R. Riordan. 1994. Phosphorylation by cAMP-dependent protein kinase causes a conformational change in the R domain of the cystic fibrosis transmembrane conductance regulator. *Biochemistry.* 33:4072–4079.

Frizzell, R. A., M. Field, and S. G. Schultz. 1979. Sodium-coupled chloride transport by epithelial tissues. *American Journal of Physiology.* 236:F1–F8.

Gadsby, D. C., and A. C. Nairn. 1994. Regulation of CFTR channel gating. *Trends in Biochemical Sciences.* 19:513–518.

Gray, M.A., A. Harris, L. Coleman, J.R. Greenwell, M.A. Gray, A. Harris, L. Coleman, J.R. Greenwell, and B.E. Argent. 1989. Two types of chloride channel on duct cells cultured from human fetal pancreas. *American Journal of Physiology.* 257:C240–C251.

Gregory, R. J., D. P. Rich, S. H. Cheng, D. W. Souza, S. Paul, P. Manavalan, M. P. Anderson, M. J. Welsh, and A. E. Smith. 1991. Maturation and function of cystic fibrosis transmembrane conductance regulator variants bearing mutations in putative nucleotide-binding domains 1 and 2. *Molecular and Cell Biology.* 11:3886–3893.

Gunderson, K. L., and R. R. Kopito. 1994. Effects of pyrophosphate and nucleotide analogs suggest a role for ATP hydrolysis in cystic fibrosis transmembrane regulator channel gating. *Journal of Biological Chemistry.* 269:19349–19353.

Halm, D.R., G. Rechkemmer, R.A. Shoumaler, and R.A. Frizzell. 1988. Biophysical properties of a chloride channel in the apical membrane of a secretory epithelial cell. *Comparative Biochemistry and Physiology.* 90A:597–601.

Hanrahan, J. W., J. A. Tabcharani, and R. Grygorczyk. 1993. Patch clamp studies of apical membrane chloride channels. *In* Cystic Fibrosis: Current Topics. Vol. 1. J. A. Dodge, D. J. H. Brock, and J. H. Widdicombe, editors. John Wiley & Sons, Inc., Chichester. 93–137

Haws, C. M., W. E. Finkbeiner, J. H. Widdicombe, and J. J. Wine. 1993. Calu-3, a model

CFTR expressing cell line: novel features of CFTR channel regulation. *Pediatric Pulmonology*. 9(Suppl.):215–216.

Hwang, T.-C., T. Baukrowitz, G. Nagel, A. C. Horie, and D. C. Gadsby. 1994. Regulation of the gating of cardiac CFTR Cl channels by phosphorylation and ATP hydrolysis. *Journal of General Physiology*. 104:34*a*. (Abstr.)

Hwang, T.-C., M. Horie, and D. C. Gadsby. 1993. Functionally distinct phospho-forms underlie incremental activation of protein kinase-regulated Cl^- conductance in mammalian heart. *Journal of General Physiology*. 101:629–650.

Hwang, T.-C., G. Nagel, A. C. Nairn, and D. C. Gadsby. 1994. Regulation of the gating of cystic fibrosis transmembrane conductance regulator Cl channels by phosphorylation and ATP hydrolysis. *Proceedings of the National Academy of Sciences*. 91:4698–4702.

Illek, B., H. Fischer, G. Santos, J. H. Widdicombe, T. E. Machen, and W. W. Reenstra. 1994. Cyclic AMP-independent activation of CFTR Cl channels by the tyrosine kinase inhibitor genistein. *Journal of General Physiology*. 104:36*a*. (Abstr.)

Kartner, N., J. W. Hanrahan, T. J. Jensen, A. L. Naismith, S. Sun, C. A. Ackerley, E. F. Reyes, L.-C. Tsui, J. M. Rommens, C. E. Bear, and J. R. Riordan. 1991. Expression of the cystic fibrosis gene in non-epithelial invertebrate cells produces a regulated anion conductance. *Cell*. 64:681–691.

Kristidis, P., D. Bozon, M. Corey, D. Markiewicz, J. Rommens, L.-C. Tsui, and P. Durie. 1992. Genetic determination of exocrine pancreatic function in cystic fibrosis. *American Journal of Human Genetics*. 50:1178–1184.

Mansoura, M. K., T. V. Strong, F. S. Collins, and D. C. Dawson. 1994. A disease-related mutation in the fifth putative transmembrane segment alters the conduction and gating properties of CFTR. *Journal of General Physiology*. 104:36*a*. (Abstr.)

McDonough, S., N. Davidson, H. A. Lester, and N. A. McCarty. 1994. Novel pore-lining residues in CFTR that govern permeation and open-channel block. *Neuron*. 13:1–20.

Nagel, G., T.-C. Hwang, K.L. Nastiuk, A.C. Nairn, and D.C. Gadsby. 1992. The protein kinase A-regulated cardiac Cl^- channel resembles the cystic fibrosis transmembrane conductance regulator. *Nature*. 360:81–84.

Oblatt-Montal, M., G. L. Reddy, T. Iwamoto, J. M. Tomich, and M. Montal. 1994. Identification of an ion channel-forming motif in the primary structure of CFTR, the cystic fibrosis chloride channel. *Proceedings of the National Academy of Sciences, USA*. 91:1495–1499.

Ostedgaard, L. S., D. N. Sheppard, and M. J. Welsh. 1994. Biochemical and functional analysis of mutations in the first nucleotide-binding domain of CFTR which are associated with pancreatic sufficiency. *Journal of General Physiology*. 104:35a–36a. (Abstr.)

Quinton, P. M. 1983. Chloride impermeability in cystic fibrosis. *Nature*. 301:421–422.

Quinton, P. M. 1990. Cystic fibrosis: a disease in electrolyte transport. *FASEB Journal*. 4:2709–2717.

Quinton, P. M., and M. M. Reddy. 1992. Control of CFTR chloride conductance by ATP levels through nonhydrolytic binding. *Nature*. 360:79–81.

Reisin, I. L., A. G. Prat, E. H. Abraham, J. F. Amara, R. J. Gregory, D. A. Ausiello, and H. F. Cantiello. 1994. The cystic fibrosis transmembrane conductance regulator is a dual ATP and chloride channel. *Journal of Biological Chemistry*. 269:20584–20591.

Riordan, J. R., J. M. Rommens, B. Kerem, N. Alon, R. Rozmahel, Z. Grzelczak, J. Zielenski, S. Lok, N. Plavsic, J.-L. Chou, M. L. Drumm, M. C. Iannuzzi, F. S. Collins, and L.-C. Tsui.

1989. Identification of the cystic fibrosis gene: cloning and characterization of complementary DNA. *Science.* 245:1066–1073.

Rommens, J. M., M. C. Iannuzzi, B. Kerem, M. L. Drumm, G. Melmer, M. Dean, R. Rozmahel, J. L. Cole, D. Kennedy, N. Hidaka, M. Zsiga, M. Buchwald, J. R. Riordan, L. Tsui, and F. S. Collins. 1989. Identication of the Cystic Fibrosis gene: chromosome walking and jumping. *Science*. 245:1059–1065.

Schaedel, C., A.-C. Kristoffersson, R. Kornfält, and L. Holmberg. 1994. A novel cystic fibrosis mutation, Y109C, in the first transmembrane domain of CFTR. *Human Molecular Genetics.* 3:1001–1002.

Sheppard, D. N., L. S. Ostedgaard, D. P. Rich, and M. J. Welsh. 1994. The amino-terminal portion of CFTR forms a regulated Cl^- channel. *Cell.* 76:1091–1098.

Seibert, F.S., J.A. Tabcharani, X.-B. Chang, A.M. Dulhanty, C.J. Mathews, J.W. Hanrahan, and J.R. Riordan. 1995. cAMP-dependent protein kinase-mediated phosphorylation of cystic fibrosis transmembrane conductance regulator residue Ser-753 and its role in channel activation. *Journal of Biological Chemistry.* 270:2158–2162.

Smit, L. S., D. J. Wilkinson, M. K. Mansoura, F. S. Collins, and D. C. Dawson. 1993. Functional roles of the nucleotide binding folds in the activation of the cystic fibrosis transmembrane conductance regulator. *Proceedings of the National Academy of Sciences, USA*. 90:9963–9967.

Tabcharani, J. A., X.-B. Chang, J. R. Riordan, and J. W. Hanrahan. 1991. Phosphorylation-regulated Cl- channel in CHO cells stably expressing the cystic fibrosis gene. *Nature.* 352:628–631.

Tabcharani, J. A., X.-B. Chang, J. R. Riordan, and J. W. Hanrahan. 1992. The cystic fibrosis transmembrane conductance regulator chloride channel. Iodide block and permeation. *Biophysical Journal.* 62:1–4.

Tabcharani, J. A., W. Low, D. Elie, and J. W. Hanrahan. 1990. Low-conductance chloride channel activated by cAMP in the epithelial cell line T_{84}. *FEBS Letters.* 270:157–164.

Tabcharani, J. A., J. M. Rommens, Y.-X. Hou, X.-B. Chang, L.-C. Tsui, J. R. Riordan, and J. W. Hanrahan. 1993. Multi-ion pore behaviour in the CFTR chloride channel. *Nature.* 366:79–82.

Tsui, L.-C. 1992. The spectrum of cystic fibrosis mutations. *Trends in Genetics*. 8:392–398.

Wagner, J. A., A. L. Cozens, H. Schulman, D. C. Gruenert, L. Stryer, and P. Gardner. 1991. Activation of chloride channels in normal and cystic fibrosis airway epithelial cells by multifunctional calcium/calmodulin-dependent protein kinase. *Nature*. 349:793–796.

Winter, M. C., D. N. Sheppard, M. R. Carson, and M. J. Welsh. 1994. Effect of ATP concentration on CFTR Cl-channels: a kinetic analysis of channel regulation. *Biophysical Journal*. 66:1398–1403.

Worrell, R. T., and R. A. Frizzell. 1991. CaMKII mediates stimulation of chloride conductance by calcium in T84 cells. *American Journal of Physiology*. 260:C877–C882.

Treatment of Cystic Fibrosis Based on Understanding CFTR

Alan E. Smith

Genzyme Corporation, Framingham, Massachusetts 01701

One of the fundamental tenets of the reductionist approach to medicine is that by gaining a molecular understanding of biological systems, we will learn not only how living organisms function but also how to utilize such information to understand and treat disease. Such a molecular approach has had success in the development of drugs that regulate metabolic processes and that control the growth of infectious organisms. With the advent of our ability to investigate human genetics at the molecular level, such a reductionist approach is now possible in the study of inherited diseases. This is perhaps nowhere more evident than current attempts to devise treatments for cystic fibrosis (CF). The gene causing the disease has been isolated and sequenced, and the gene product has been identified and characterized. The function of the gene product has been elucidated. Hundreds of mutations associated with the disease have been identified and in many cases, the effects of the mutation upon the gene product and on its function have been established. Gene knock-outs to produce a variety of CF mice has been accomplished. Not only is the disease well understood, the disease is common, patients are well organized and motivated and specific funding agencies that enthusiastically and generously support research on the disease exist worldwide. The purpose of this review is to summarize progress towards devising a treatment for CF based on a molecular understanding of the disease gained in the five years since the gene was isolated.

Cystic Fibrosis Disease

CF is a disease affecting epithelia in a variety of tissues including sweat ducts, pancreas, reproductive tissues and especially pulmonary airways (Boat, Welsh, and Beaudet, 1989). The characteristic dysfunction is in the movement of salt and water across affected epithelia. The consequences of this vary with tissue, but in general, they are not life threatening given good patient care. The exception to this is disease in the pulmonary airways. In this case there are changes in the composition of mucus secretions which lead to defective mucociliary clearance. Patients usually succumb to bacterial infection, commonly with *psuedomonas auroginosa,* setting in motion a cycle of inflammation, tissue damage, impaired lung function and eventually death. Median survival in the United States is ~29 yr.

CFTR, the CF Gene Product

For a detailed description of the CF gene and its gene product (called CFTR) readers are referred to recent reviews (Riordan, 1993; Welsh, Anderson, Rich, Berger, Denning, Ostegaard, Sheppard, Cheng, Gregory, and Smith, 1992). In summary, CFTR is a glycosylated, integral membrane protein of 1,480 amino acids, belonging to a broad class of polypeptides referred to as ABC- or ATP-dependent transporters. The protein comprises two copies of a membrane spanning domain containing six transmembrane sequences, two copies of a nucleotide binding domain and a single copy of a regulatory or R domain (Riordan, 1993).

CFTR functions as a chloride channel, controlled by phosphorylation of a number of sites within the R domain, and by the binding of nucleotides within the nucleotide binding folds. The transmembrane domains appear to form a channel through which chloride passes (Welsh et al., 1992). Four classes of mutations associated with CF and resulting in CFTR dysfunction have been described (Welsh and Smith, 1993). The most common class of mutation (II), typified by the ΔF508 mutation, results in CFTR that is defective in intracellular trafficking from endoplasmic reticulum to golgi (Cheng, Gregory, Marshall, Paul, Souza, White, Riordan, and Smith, 1990). Interestingly, some mutations in the transmembrane regions cause only relatively minor purturbation to CFTR chloride conductance and are associated with only mild CF disease (Sheppard, et al., 1993). Other than this, knowledge of the genotype does not yet allow meaningful predictions of disease outcome.

Molecular Approaches to Treatment of CF Disease

Based on information acquired since the discovery of the CF gene, it is possible to devise approaches to the disease that attempt to correct the newly characterized molecular defects. Such approaches include attempts to (*a*) regulate transepithelial salt balance, particularly movement of chloride ions; (*b*) move variant CFTR molecules with a trafficking defect to the correct cellular location; (*c*) augment the defective CFTR protein by delivery of recombinant CFTR; and (*d*) augment the defective CFTR gene by delivery of the wild-type DNA sequence. Because lung disease is the most life threatening aspect of CF, most present efforts focus to this tissue to develop such approaches.

Regulation of Transepithelial Salt Balance

This approach is perhaps the least impacted by cloning of the CF gene because the defect in salt balance was well characterized before knowledge of the protein responsible. Indeed, pharmacological studies seeking agents to ameliorate the disease state by restoring the salt and water balance across airway epithelia predate cloning of the CF gene. Although we now know that the defect is a direct result of dysfunction of CFTR, presumably because of abnormal chloride transport, it is not obvious how this leads to abnormal sodium transport.

Activation of alternative chloride channels. Human airway epithelial cells contain chloride channels other than CFTR. A screening of compounds able to activate such alternative channels showed that ATP and UTP had such activity probably by activating a purinergic receptor (Knowles, Clarke, and Boucher, 1991). Preclinical studies suggested that UTP was preferable to ATP and limited trials of UTP are underway.

Amiloride. Amiloride is a diuretic active in regulating sodium transport. By decreasing the abnormally high sodium absorption observed in CF epithelia, it was predicted that lung function might improve. Early clinical trials of repeated dosing of aerosolized amiloride to test this hypothesis appear promising (Knowles, Church, Waltner, Yankaskas, Gilligan, King, Edwards, Helms, and Boucher, 1990).

Restoration of Trafficking of Mutant CFTR

The recognition that several mutant versions of CFTR, including the most common ΔF508 mutation, have a trafficking defect suggests a completely new approach to treatment of CF; the development of drugs able to facilitate movement of CFTR variants that otherwise fail to traffic correctly (Cheng et al., 1990; Welsh and Smith, 1993). Such an approach would only be of value if the variant CFTR retained at least some chloride channel activity. Two general approaches can be taken, one is to intervene in the trafficking process itself, the other relies on overexpression of mutant CFTR.

CFTR transcription. When overexpressed in recombinant cells, a fraction of ΔF508 CFTR appears able to override the defect and traffic correctly and, because the mutant retains some basal activity, increased chloride channel activity can be detected. Screening of agents able to regulate CFTR expression has shown that the most effective compound detected so far is sodium butyrate (Smith, unpublished results). This agent has the ability to stimulate transcription of a variety of genes. For example, currently it is in clinical trials for the treatment of thalasemia where it is hoped it will stimulate transcription of fetal globin genes and thereby overcome the lack of adult globin. At present, although CFTR activity appears to be enhanced by butyrate treatment of CF cells in culture, it has not been possible to correct CF epithelia in monolayer culture. More potent and/or more specific reagents may be required before testing for clinical efficacy is warranted.

CFTR chaperones. The mechanism whereby normal CFTR moves through the cell remains unclear. It is likely that CFTR variants with a trafficking defect are unable to fold correctly and that the misfolded protein is recognized by a so-called quality control mechanism located within the endoplasmic reticulum. What is recognized as abnormal by the quality control mechanism is not known. It has been claimed that CFTR interacts with the chaperones calnexin and hsp70 but there are no reports of inhibitors of these interactions. At this stage, it is not known whether it will be possible to develop drugs that specifically inhibit trafficking of individual proteins without more generalized toxic effects on the synthesis of a broader spectrum of cellular proteins.

Augment Defective CFTR Protein

Protein replacement therapy for genetic diseases involves administration of the protein product of the defective gene. For example, blood products are used to treat various hemoglobinopathies and glucocerebrosidase to treat Gaucher's disease. Clearly, such an approach to treat CF is technically more challenging than the systemic administration of a soluble blood protein.

Recombinant insect cells have been developed that produce large amounts of active CFTR. The protein has also been produced in recombinant CHO cells and in the milk of transgenic mice. The feasibility of CFTR delivery has been demonstrated using CFTR purified from both CHO and insect cells. The protein was incorporated into liposomes including influenza HA as a fusogen or into influenza virosomes. Fusion to recipient cells was brought about by brief treatment with low pH to activate the HA molecules. Evidence of insertion of CFTR into the recipient membrane was obtained by assaying for CFTR function using a fluorescent dye that is quenched by iodide ions. Exit of iodide via the introduced CFTR molecules lead to increased fluorescence upon activation by cAMP (unpublished results). Although these experiments appear to demonstrate correct introduction of active CFTR into cells in culture, additional data demonstrating transfer of the protein by other analytical methods and transfer into epithelial monolayers would be desirable.

Augment Defective CF Gene

At present, much emphasis is being placed on gene therapy approaches to CF. One reason for this is that such treatment has the potential to address the fundamental disease state (Mulligan, 1993). For CF, the initial disease target is the airway epithelium. Cells in this tissue turn over relatively slowly. This immediately suggests that treatment will very likely need to be in vivo because airway cells cannot be replaced readily and involve vectors other than retroviruses since these require dividing cells. By contrast, most experience to date in gene therapy has involved ex vivo treatment, using retroviruses.

Viral versus nonviral systems. That early attempts at gene therapy for any disease should involve vectors based on viruses is very predictable (Mulligan, 1993). Viruses function to bring about the transfer of nucleic acids to different cells, they are relatively simple to manipulate in the laboratory and selection pressure over millions of years has ensured that viruses are very efficient. However, viral vectors raise a variety of potential safety issues. The alternative is to argue that gene therapy requires a synthetic approach, such as the use of cationic lipids (Felgner, Kumar, Stridhar, Wheeler, Tsai, Border, Ramsey, Martin, and Felgner, 1994), where the ease of manufacture and especially the safety profile is likely to be very much more favorable. The difficulty of this approach is that the efficacy of gene transfer is much lower.

At present, there is insufficient data to conclude whether a viral or nonviral approach is best for use in CF. In the end, it seems likely that a synthesis of both approaches will occur. Viral genes will continually be removed to generate an entity looking less and less like a virus whereas components, perhaps from viruses, will be added to nonviral systems in any attempt to improve their efficacy.

Adenovirus-based vectors. Adenoviruses have provided the first viral vector system for CF (Rosenfeld et al., 1992; Zabner et al., 1994). These are relatively small double stranded DNA viruses associated in general with mild disease. Strains of the virus naturally infect airway cells. The molecular biology of the virus is well understood (Berkner, 1988; Graham and Prevec, 1992). All adenovirus based vectors presently under investigation for treatment of CF have some common features. All are E1 replacement vectors that disable the vector by removal of most of the crucial E1 region. All rely for vector growth on the 293 cell line, a human cell constitutively expressing the human Ad5 E1 region proteins and able to complement the growth of E1 deficient viruses. However, of the viruses reported to date, significant differences also exist. A variety of different promoters are used to express CFTR sequences, different polyadenylation sequences are employed, some vectors are based on Ad2, most on Ad5. Perhaps the most significant difference is that most vectors delete the viral E3 region whereas some do not. The E3 region is dispensable for viral growth in cell culture and its removal generates more space in the viral genome for exogenous DNA sequences. E3, however, codes for a number of viral functions, most of which are involved in generating resistance to defense mechanisms normally mounted to rid the host of infectious organisms (Ginsberg, Lundholm-Beauchamp, Horswood, Pernis, Wold, Chanock, and Prince, 1989). These include gene products conferring resistance to TNF-α and in blunting the host MHC class 1-based immune response. These properties, if expressed, would be expected to reduce the host response to added vector.

β-galactosidase encoding vectors are often used to examine gene delivery. Such studies using adenovirus based vectors have shown that delivery to the lung of rats, primates and mice is quite efficient with a high proportion of cells expressing enzyme after administration of a modest number of infectious units per cell. Infection of a variety of cell types appears possible. Results of experiments to determine the duration of expression and the efficacy of repeated dosing vary. Nevertheless, there is a general expectation that vector expression will not persist long enough to obviate repeat dosing.

Initial reports on the safety profile of E1 replacement adenovirus vectors in rodents and primates reported different degrees of pathology associated with vector administration. Some reports suggested very little inflammation in cotton rats and rhesus monkeys, others reported more severe inflammation, particularly in alveolar regions after administration to a baboon (Zabner et al., 1994; Simon et al., 1993). These differences have lead to more systematic studies, many in mice where the process of inflammation, particularly the role of the immune system, can be evaluated in detail. At present some inflammation has been detected with most vectors tested. The effect is clearly dose dependent. There appear to be differences in sensitivity between species and between mouse strains. Earlier reports using wild-type adenovirus, showed that administration results in two phases of inflammation; an early phase characterized by the appearance of the cytokines IL-1, IL-6, and TNF and of monocyte/macrophage cells and a later phase characterized by the appearance of lymphocytes (Ginsberg, Moldawer, Sehgal, Redington, Kilian, Chancock, and Prince, 1991). These studies suggest that the later phase of inflammation is caused by development of cytotoxic T lymphocytes (CTL) directed against viral proteins. More recent studies with E1 replacement vectors claim that CTL also develop and that these CTLs destroy cells expressing the introduced gene, thereby reducing the duration of expression (Yang, Nunes, Berencsi, Furth, Gonczol, and Wilson, 1994).

AAV vectors. AAV is a very small single stranded human DNA virus with apparently no associated pathology. The vector is easy to manipulate and again has the ability to infect human airway cells. AAV has the advantage that it is capable of integrating into the host cell chromosome at least under some circumstances (Muzyczka, 1994).

The current limitations on the use of AAV vectors are twofold. First, the size of the genome of AAV is limited. Because the size of the minimal wild-type CFTR cDNA exceeds the optimal size of an AAV vector insert, it is difficult to generate an efficient CFTR vector and retain the ability to package efficiently. Second, growth of AAV vectors requires introduction into cells of two plasmids: the vector containing the gene of interest and terminal repeats plus a helper vector encoding *cap* and *env* required for AAV replication as well as superinfection with adeno or other helper virus. This procedure is cumbersome and presently yields amounts of virus insufficient for large scale animal studies.

A wide variety of approaches are being taken to avoid these problems. These include reducing the size of the coding sequence and regulatory elements to a minimum, and generating a variety of AAV packaging cell lines. Some studies involving administration of AAV to rabbits and to primates have been reported (Flotte, Afione, Conrad, McGrath, Solow, Oka, Zeitlin, Guggino, and Carter, 1994).

Cationic lipids. A variety of cationic lipids are now known that have the ability to complex with DNA and aid its entry into cells in culture. The mechanism whereby this occurs is unclear. The efficiency with which cationic lipids aid gene transfer into different cells grown in culture varies but in some cases it can be high, meaning virtually all cells express detectable gene product (Felgner et al., 1994).

Recent reports have generated much interest in the use of cationic lipids for CF gene therapy. First, the claim that a single dose of complex either by aerosol or by intravenous administration lead to high level, long lived expression (Zhu, Liggitt, Liu, and Debs, 1993). Second, the claim that it is possible to correct the defect in epithelial cell voltage in CF mice by administration of cationic lipid DNA complexes (Hyde, Gill, Higgins, Trezise, MacVinish, Cuthbert, Ratcliff, Evans, and Colledge, 1993). Although these results are controversial, they illustrate the potential utility of cationic lipid complexes. However, expression in most reports is transient and most investigators report a wide range of variability in the effects measured, say in individual animals. This implies some aspects of the use of cationic lipid complexes is not yet understood or optimized. Systematic studies to optimize the use of these reagents, particularly in animals, are required before it will be possible to assess the potential of cationic lipids for gene transfer for CF.

Molecular conjugates. This term refers to complexes made containing the DNA of interest and any number of additional molecules designed to assist entry of DNA into the cell. Most complexes in this category contain polylysine as an agent to condense the DNA and neutralize its charge. In addition, a ligand is usually added to aid entry into the cell by receptor-mediated endocytosis.

For airway applications, two ligands have been used, antibody to the polymeric IgA receptor and surfactant proteins (Ferkol, Kaetzel, and Davis, 1993). Other studies have utilized a ubiquitous ligand such as transferin. One problem encountered in many studies is the ability of the DNA once inside the cell to escape from the endosome. Because adenovirus has a well characterized ability to escape endosomes, one approach has been to conjugate adenovirus to a ligand:polylysine:DNA complex. Large increases in transfection efficacy have been reported at least in cell culture using this approach (Curiel, Wagner, Cotten, Birnstiel, Li, Loechel, Agarwal, and Hu, 1994). However, the use of such conjugates in vivo appear more problematic.

As with the cationic lipids, the efficacy and duration of expression appear key issues that require improvement before molecular conjugates become as efficient as viruses. The dilemma, of course, is that as each additional component is added to a molecular conjugate to improve its efficacy, its size, complexity, and potential toxicity also increases. Whether efficiency can be improved to a greater extent than these undesirable properties remains unknown, but it should not go unnoticed that the selection pressures that have driven the evolution of viruses are lacking in laboratory attempts to assemble efficient complexes. It requires a great deal of our creativity to build an effective molecular conjugage starting from first principles.

Clinical data. Given that it is impossible to predict, based on animal experiments, the likely clinical utility of the various alternative gene therapy vectors that are presently available, early testing of some of them in CF patients appears justified provided an acceptable benefit to risk analysis can be argued.

Three tissues are presently targeted. The nasal epithelium, the maxillary sinus and airway epithelium. The nasal protocols attempt to gain safety data on viral administration as well as evidence of electrophysiological correction of the CF defect, whereas at the same time minimizing risk to the patient. In one study, treatment of three patients demonstrated a measurable change in transepithelial voltage after administration of Ad2/CFTR-1. No evidence of viral replication or of virus associated inflammation was obtained (Zabner et al., 1993). This study is being followed by a repeat dose, dose escalation safety study in the nose and an attempt to gain evidence of changed biological parameters such as bacterial load, cytokine profile and MRI after repeat dosing of Ad2/CFTR-2 to the sinus. Other protocols have administered increasing doses of adenovirus vector by bronchoscope to a segment of the lung. Although not published, one of these studies encountered an adverse reaction in a patient at a dose of 2×10^9 infectious units. These continuing safety studies are important because they hopefully will define whether a therapeutic window exists within which the likely benefits of gene therapy can be assessed without exposing the patient to unacceptable risks. Further, such studies will help to define characteristics of the adenovirus vector that require improvement based on human rather than animal data.

A recent lipid based nasal administration protocol was completed in London. These results are unpublished but reports indicate success in correcting transepithelial voltage was limited but encouraging. The safety profile was good.

Conclusions

Progress in understanding the basic defect in CF has proceeded at great speed and with much fanfare over the last five years. It is clear that our understanding of the gene, the gene product and its function has increased immeasurably. That this knowledge suggests new approaches to treatment of the disease is also unquestionable. When and how this translates into improved therapies remains the question. What is required is an effective treatment, not necessarily one that is scientifically elegant or a technical tour-de-force. This argues that it is important to continue research into various approaches to the disease and not to decide on theoretic grounds that one approach is superior. What appears scientifically most straight forward may not be the most practicable. At this stage, however, in spite of the practical problems that need to be overcome before an effective treatment becomes available, it is difficult not to be optimistic about the prospects for improved therapy.

References

Berkner, K. L. 1988. Development of adenovirus vectors for the expression of heterologous genes. *Biotechniques.* 6:616–629.

Boat, T. F., M. J. Welsh, and A. L. Beaudet. 1989. Cystic fibrosis. *In* The Metabolic Basis of Inherited Disease. C. R. Scriver, A. L. Beaudet, W. S. Sly, and D. Valle, editors. McGraw-Hill, Inc., New York, NY. 2649–2680.

Cheng, S. H., R. J. Gregory, J. Marshall, S. Paul, D. W. Souza, G. A. White, C. R. O'Riordan, and A. E. Smith. 1990. Defective intracellular transport and processing of CFTR is the molecular basis of most cystic fibrosis. *Cell.* 63:827–834.

Curiel, D. T., E. Wagner, M. Cotten, M. L. Birnstiel, C.-M. Li, S. Loechel, S. Agarwal, and P.-C. Hu. 1992. High efficiency gene transfer medited by adenovirus coupled to DNA-polylysine complexes. *Human Gene Therapy.* 3:147–154.

Felgner, J. H., C. N. Kumar, C. N. Stridhar, C. J. Wheeler, Y. J. Tsai, R. Border, P. Ramsey, M. Martin, and P. L. Felgner. 1994. Enhanced gene delivery and mechanism studies with a novel series of cationic lipid formulations. *Journal of Biological Chemistry.* 269:2550–2561.

Ferkol, T., C. S. Kaetzel, and P. B. Davis. 1993. Gene transfer into respiratory epithelial cells by targeting the polymeric immunoglobulin receptor. *Journal of Clinical Investigation.* 92:2394–2400.

Flotte, T. R., S. A. Afione, C. Conrad, S. A. McGrath, R. Solow, H. Oka, P. L. Zeitlin, W. B. Guggino, and B. J. Carter. 1993. Stable in vivo expression of the cystic fibrosis transmembrane conductance regulator with an adeno-associated virus vector. *Proceedings of the National Academy of Sciences, USA.* 90:10613–10617.

Ginsberg, H. S., L. L. Moldawer, P. B. Sehgal, M. Redington, P. L. Kilian, R. M. Chancock, and G. A. Prince. 1991. A mouse model for investigating the molecular pathogenesis of adenovirus pneumonia. *Proceedings of the National Academy of Sciences, USA.* 88:1651–1655.

Ginsberg, H. S., U. Lundholm-Beauchamp, R. L. Horswood, B. Pernis, W. S. Wold, R. M. Chanock, and G. A. Prince. 1989. Role of early region 3 (E3) in pathogenesis of adenovirus disease. *Proceedings of the National Academy of Sciences, USA.* 86:3823–3827.

Graham, F. L., and L. Prevec. 1992. Adenovirus-based expression vectors and recombinant vaccines. *In* Vaccines: New Approaches to Immunological Problems. R. W. Ellis, editor. Butterworth-Heinemann, Boston. 363–390.

Hyde, S. C., D. R. Gill, C. F. Higgins, A. E. Trezise, L. J. MacVinish, A. W. Cuthbert, R. Ratcliff, M. J. Evans, and W. H. Colledge. 1993. Correction of the ion transport defect in cystic fibrosis transgenic mice by gene therapy. *Nature.* 362:250–255.

Knowles, M. R., L. L. Clarke, and R. C. Boucher. 1991. Activation by extracellular nucleotides of chloride secretion in the airway epithelia of patients with cystic fibrosis. *New England Journal of Medicine.* 325:533–538.

Knowles, M. R., N. L. Church, W. E. Waltner, J. R. Yankaskas, P. Gilligan, M. King, L. J. Edwards, R. W. Helms, and R. C. Boucher. 1990. A pilot study of aerosolized amiloride for the treatment of lung disease in cystic fibrosis. *New England Journal of Medicine.* 322:1189–1194.

Mulligan, R. C. 1993. The basic science of gene therapy. *Science.* 260:926–932.

Muzyczka, N. 1992. Current Topic in Microbiology and Immunology. Springer-Verlag, Berlin. 97–129.

Riordan, J. R. 1993. The cystic fibrosis transmembrane conductance regulator. *Annual Review of Physiology.* 55:609–630.

Rosenfeld, M. A., K. Yoshimura, B. C. Trapnell, K. Yoneyama, E. R. Rosenthal, W. Dalemans, M. Fukayama, J. Bargon, L. E. Stier, L. Stratford-Perricaudet, M. Perricaudet, W. B. Guggino, A. Pavirani, J-P. Lecocq, and R. G. Crystal. 1992. In vivo transfer of the human cystic fibrosis transmembrane conductance regulator gene to the airway epithelium. *Cell.* 68:143–155.

Sheppard, D. N., D. P. Rich, L. S. Ostedgaard, R. J. Gregory, A. E. Smith, and M. J. Welsh. 1993. Mutations in CFTR associated with mild disease form Cl^- channels with altered pore properties. *Nature.* 362:160–164.

Simon, R. H., J. F. Engelhardt, Y. Yang, M. Zepeda, S. W. Pendleton, M. Grossman, and J. M. Wilson. 1993. Adenovirus-mediated transfer of the CFTR gene to lung of nonhuman primates: toxicity study. 4:771–780.

Welsh, M. J., and A. E. Smith. 1993. Molecular mechanisms of CFTR chloride channel dysfunction in cystic fibrosis. *Cell.* 73:1251–1254.

Welsh, M. J., M. P. Anderson, D. P. Rich, H. A. Berger, G. M. Denning, L. S. Ostedgaard, D. N. Sheppard, S. H. Cheng, R. J. Gregory, and A. E. Smith. 1992. Cystic fibrosis transmembrane conductance regulator: a chloride channel with novel regulation. *Neuron.* 8:821–829.

Yang, Y., F. A. Nunes, K. Berencsi, E. E. Furth, E. Gonczol, and J. M. Wilson. 1994. Cellular immunity to viral antigens limits E1-deleted adenoviruses for gene therapy. *Proceedings of the National Academy of Sciences, USA.* 91:6196–6200.

Zabner, J., L. A. Couture, R. J. Gregory, S. M. Graham, A. E. Smith, and M. J. Welsh. 1993. Adenovirus-mediated gene transfer transiently corrects the chloride transport defect in patients with cystic fibrosis. *Cell.* 75:207–216.

Zabner, J., D. M. Petersen, A. P. Puga, S. M. Graham, L. A. Couture, L. D. Keyes, M. J. Lukason, J. A. St George, R. J. Gregory, A. E. Smith et al. 1994. Safety and efficacy of repetitive adenovirus-mediated transfer of CFTR cDNA to airway epithelia of primates and cotton rats. *Nature Genetics.* 6:75–83.

Zhu, N., D. Liggitt, Y. Liu, and R. Debs. 1993. Systemic gene expression after intravenous DNA delivery into adult mice. *Science.* 261:209–211.

Myotonias due to CLC-1 Chloride Channel Mutations

Thomas J. Jentsch, Claudius Lorenz, Michael Pusch, and Klaus Steinmeyer

Center for Molecular Neurobiology (ZMNH), Hamburg University, D-20246 Hamburg, Germany

Myotonia is characterized by an impairment of muscle relaxation after voluntary contraction and is due to an electrical instability of the muscle plasma membrane (for review, see Rüdel and Lehmann-Horn, 1985). This leads to a train of action potentials after a single stimulus (myotonic runs). In myotonic dystrophy, which has several other symptoms in addition to myotonia, the product of the mutated gene is probably a protein kinase (Fu et al., 1992; Mahadevan et al., 1992; Brook et al., 1992). The mechanism by which it leads to myotonia, however, is presently unclear. Another form of myotonia can be precipitated by exposure to cold temperatures (paramyotonia congenita). It is now known that this disease, as well as hyperkalemic periodic paralysis, are due to mutations in the skeletal muscle sodium channel (Fontaine et al., 1990; Rojas, Wang, Schwartz, Hoffman, Powell, and Brown, 1991; McClatchey et al., 1992). These mutations lead to defects in channel inactivation. This produces late sodium currents which depolarize the membrane, leading in turn to myotonic runs. In being due to gain-of-function mutations, both paramyotonia congenita as well as hyperkalemic periodic paralysis are dominant diseases.

Other forms of myotonia have now been proven to be due to mutations in the skeletal muscle chloride channel ClC-1. Both a dominant (Thomsen type) (Thomsen, 1876) and a recessive (Becker type; Becker, 1977) form of chloride channel myotonia exist. The pioneering studies of S. H. Bryant and colleagues were the first ones to indicate that chloride conductance is defective both in a myotonic goat animal model and in human patients (Lipicky and Bryant, 1966; Lipicky, Bryant, and Salmon, 1971; Bryant and Morales-Aguilera, 1971; Adrian and Bryant, 1974). Other studies confirmed these observations, and also hinted at a role of sodium channels (Rüdel, Ricker, and Lehmann-Horn, 1988; Iaizzo, Franke, Hatt, Spittelmeister, Ricker, Rüdel, and Lehmann-Horn, 1991; Franke, Iaizzo, Hatt, Spittelmeister, Ricker, and Lehmann-Horn, 1991). Recently, the cloning of the ClC-1 chloride channel (Steinmeyer et al., 1991*a*) has allowed us and others to test this hypothesis, and has provided a wealth of information on this channel and its role in myotonia. In this article, we will review our current understanding of chloride channel myotonia.

In skeletal muscle, chloride conductance is unusually high and accounts for ~80% of resting conductance. Because the equilibrium potential for chloride is close to the resting potential of the muscle cell membrane, it has a stabilizing effect on membrane potential and thus performs a role similar to that of potassium conductance in most other cells. Chloride conductance contributes significantly to the repolarization of muscle action potentials and is thus essential for the electrical stability of the muscle fiber. When inhibitors of muscle chloride channels such as

9-anthracene-carboxylic acid (9-AC) are applied to muscle fibers in vitro, large series of action potentials can be evoked by a single stimulus. This resembles the myotonic runs seen in patients with myotonia, and which are the physiological basis for the impairment of muscle relaxation in these diseases.

For a long time, voltage-dependent chloride channels have escaped biochemical and molecular characterization because there is no high-affinity inhibitor for these channels available. The expression cloning of the voltage-dependent chloride channel ClC-0 from *Torpedo* electric organ (Jentsch, Steinmeyer, and Schwarz, 1990) has led to the identification of a presumably large gene family of chloride channels (Jentsch, 1994). The first mammalian voltage-dependent chloride channel to be cloned by homology to ClC-0 was ClC-1, the major skeletal muscle chloride channel (Steinmeyer, Ortland, and Jentsch, 1991*a*). This was not surprising as the electric organ is ontogenetically derived from skeletal muscle. ClC-1 is ~50% identical in amino-acid sequence to the *Torpedo* channel and shares the same transmembrane topology (Fig. 1). We assume that these channel proteins have ~12 transmembrane domains. However, this model is hypothetical as it is based mainly on simple hydropathy analysis. In fact, our initial model (Jentsch et al., 1990) had to be modified to account for results obtained with mutagenesis studies (Gründer, Thiemann, Pusch, and Jentsch, 1992) on ClC-2, a ubiquitously expressed swelling-activated chloride channel (Thiemann et al., 1992). Moreover, recent glycosylation studies demonstrate that the segment between domains D8 and D9 is glycosylated in the ClC-K kidney chloride channels (Kieferle, Fong, Bens, Vandewalle, and Jentsch, 1994) as well as in ClC-0 (Middleton, Pheasant, and Miller, 1994). This places this segment in the extracellular space. The electrophysiological properties of ClC-1 are quite different from those of ClC-0. While both channels share a chloride over bromide ion selectivity, a block by iodide, and a fast gate opening the channel upon depolarization, ClC-0 also has another (slow) gate opening the channel upon hyperpolarization. ClC-0 has a single-channel conductance of ~9 pS (Miller and White, 1984; Bauer, Steinmeyer, Schwarz, and Jentsch, 1991). In contrast, the mammalian muscle channel ClC-1 has a much lower conductance of ~1 pS which can only be measured by noise analysis (Pusch, Steinmeyer, and Jentsch, 1994). This very low single-channel conductance is sufficient to explain why studies aimed at characterizing the main muscle chloride channel at the single-channel level have invariably failed.

Ion selectivity, voltage dependence, and pharmacology (inhibition by 9-AC) agree very well with data obtained previously for macroscopic muscle chloride conductance (Palade and Barchi, 1977), suggesting that ClC-1 may indeed be the major skeletal muscle chloride channel. This is also supported by the fact that its mRNA increases steeply during the first few weeks after birth in rodents, as this parallels the observed increase in muscle chloride conductance during this time (Conte Camerino, DeLuca, Mambrini, and Vrbovà, 1989). Moreover, both chloride conductance (Camerino and Bryant, 1976) as well as ClC-1 mRNA levels decrease after denervation (Klocke, Steinmeyer, Jentsch, and Jockusch, 1994). Thus, these data already strongly suggest that ClC-1 mediates the major part of muscle chloride conductance.

Genetic evidence that mutations in ClC-1 can cause myotonia was obtained at first for an animal model. There are several mouse strains which show myotonic symptoms (ADR, *adr*^{mto}, *adr*^{K}). In contrast to the myotonic goat (Bryant and Morales-Aguilera, 1971; Adrian and Bryant, 1974), myotonia in mice is inherited in an autosomal recessive fashion. By interbreeding of these mice, it was shown that the defect is allelic. The ADR strain had been most thoroughly characterized by the group of H. Jockusch (Reininghaus, Füchtbauer, Bertram, and Jockusch, 1988; Mehrke, Brinkmeier, and Jockusch, 1988), who found a significant decrease of

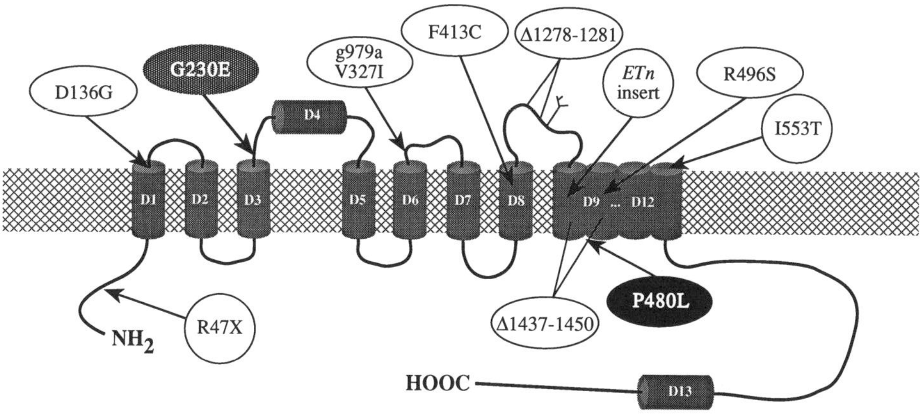

Figure 1. Location of mutations in ClC-1 leading to myotonia. Mutations in the mouse system are shown in circles, while human mutations are shown in ellipses. Recessive mutations are shown in open symbols, the fully dominant one with a black, and the partially dominant one with a hatched filling. Upper case letters indicate amino acids, whereas lower case letters refer to nucleotides. Deletions at the nucleotide level are indicated by a Δ followed by the numbers of the bases deleted (this is in part arbitrary). *ETn* insert refers to the insertion of a transposon observed in the ADR mouse (Steinmeyer et al., 1991*b*), while the two other mouse mutants have been described by Gronemeier et al. (1994) (R47X for *adr*^{mto}, and I553T for *adr*^{K}). The human recessive mutations have been found by Koch et al. (1992) (F413C), Lorenz et al. (1994) (R496S, and g979a, which affects a splice consensus site), Meyer-Kleine et al. (1994) (deletion Δ1437–1450), and Heine et al. (1994) (D136G and deletion Δ1278–1281). By shifting the reading frame, these deletions lead to stop codons in a region also affected by the *ETn* insertion of the ADR mouse. The fully dominant mutation of Dr. Thomsen's own family (P480L) was described by Steinmeyer et al. (1994). G230E, which can behave as a dominant or a recessive mutation, was found by George et al. (1993) and was functionally analyzed by Steinmeyer et al. (1994).

The topological model shown differs from previous ones (Jentsch et al., 1990; Gründer et al., 1992) as recent glycosylation studies (Kieferle et al., 1994; Middleton et al., 1994) put the region after D9 into the extracellular compartment. We propose that therefore, D4, which is not very hydrophobic and is not highly conserved in the ClC family does not cross the membrane, although this is also purely hypothetical. We do not know the topology of the D9–D12 region, which has to cross the membrane $2n + 1$ times.

muscle chloride conductance. After ClC-1 had been cloned, genomic analysis of ADR mice quickly pointed to a defect in ClC-1 as Southern analysis showed a gross abnormality of its gene. cDNA cloning then demonstrated that a transposon of the *ETn* family had inserted into an intron of ClC-1, leading to several nonfunctional transcripts (Steinmeyer, Klocke, Ortland, Gronemeier, Jockusch, Gründer, and Jentsch, 1991*b*). Interestingly, a defect in T cell development of another mouse mutant (*lpr*) was recently found to be caused by the insertion of an *ETn* transposon as well (Adachi, Watanabe-Fukunaga, and Nagata, 1993). Thus, this mutational mechanism may be quite common in mice. The ADR mouse provided unequivocal evidence that ClC-1 is essential for muscle membrane electrical stability, and that its functional destruction leads to myotonia. No gross abnormality in the ClC-1 gene could be detected by Southern analysis in other myotonic mouse strains (Steinmeyer et al., 1991*b*). Recent analysis shows that these strains carry ClC-1 point mutations (Gronemeier, Condie, Prosser, Steinmeyer, Jentsch, and Jockusch, 1994) (Fig. 1). While a stop codon before the first transmembrane domain in adr^{mto} immediately demonstrates that the gene product is nonfunctional, more detailed analysis will be necessary to demonstrate how the missense mutation in adr^{K} mice affects ClC-1 channel function. Interestingly, as expected from the increase in ClC-1 mRNA levels after birth (Steinmeyer et al., 1991*a*), myotonia in ADR mice becomes fully apparent only after more than a week, when the lack of the ClC-1 gene product is expected to gain in impact (Wischmeyer, Nolte, Klocke, Jockusch, and Brinkmeier, 1993). This also indicates that other channels dampen muscle excitability shortly after birth.

Subsequently, human ClC-1 was cloned at the cDNA and genomic levels (Koch et al., 1992; Steinmeyer, Lorenz, Pusch, Koch, and Jentsch, 1994; Lorenz, Meyer-Kleine, Steinmeyer, Koch, and Jentsch, 1994) and the corresponding gene locus (named CLCN1) located on human chromosome 7q35 (Koch et al., 1992) close to the T cell receptor beta gene (Koch et al., 1992), which is also closely linked to the *Clc-1* locus in the mouse (Steinmeyer et al., 1991*b*). The human ClC-1 gene is interrupted by 22 introns (Lorenz et al., 1994) and oligonucleotide primers now allow PCR-amplification of every single exon to search for mutations. Three restriction enzymes (*Nsi*I, *Ava*II, and *Sau*96I) detect polymorphisms in this gene in the Caucasian population (Koch et al., 1992, 1993).

While all known myotonic mouse strains show a recessive pattern of inheritance, in humans, both autosomal recessive (Becker, 1977) and dominant (Thomsen, 1876) forms of myotonia exist. Both forms of myotonia were linked to the CLCN1 locus (Koch et al., 1992) in German families, and Canadian families with dominant myotonia were linked to the nearby TCRB locus (Abdalla, Casley, Cousin, Hudson, Murphy, Cornélis, Hashimoto, and Ebers, 1992). Together with the results obtained for ADR mice, this provided very strong evidence that ClC-1 mutations are also responsible for myotonia in humans.

The first mutation identified in human myotonia was a point mutation in a German family with recessive generalized myotonia (Becker type) (Koch et al., 1992). It exchanges a highly conserved phenylalanine in putative transmembrane domain D8 for a cysteine. This mutation has now been identified in ~15% of German families with Becker type myotonia (Koch et al., 1993). Several new point mutations (Lorenz et al., 1994; Heine, George, Pika, Deymeer, Rüdel, and Lehmann-Horn, 1994) as well as short deletions (Meyer-Kleine, Ricker, Otto, and Koch, 1994; Heine et al., 1994) have recently been identified in recessive (Becker-type) myotonia. One of the point mutations occurs at an exon-intron boundary and may lead to abnormal splicing (Lorenz et al., 1994).

Different point mutations were identified in patients having dominant myotonia congenita (Thomsen's disease) (George, Crackower, Abdalla, Hudson, and Ebers,

1993; Steinmeyer et al., 1994). Dr. Thomsen, who first described the disease in 1876 (Thomsen, 1876), was affected himself. The availability of living members of his family allowed us to identify and functionally analyze the mutation (P480L) which caused myotonia in Dr. Thomsen himself (Steinmeyer et al., 1994).

How can one explain that certain mutations in the same gene lead to recessive, while others lead to dominant disease? A loss-of-function mutation, such as a missing channel protein with the early stop codon in the adr^{mto} mouse, will probably reduce muscle chloride conductance to ~50% in a heterozygote. Thus, one would have to postulate that this level of conductance is still sufficient to ensure muscle membrane stability, resulting in no overt phenotype. In vitro studies using inhibitors to block muscle chloride conductance indeed demonstrated that >50% of the chloride conductance needs to be blocked to produce myotonic runs (Kwiecinski, Lehmann-Horn, and Rüdel, 1988). In this respect, it is interesting to note that more sophisticated analysis (such as electromyograms) may be able to detect heterozygotes in families with recessive generalized myotonia (Becker, 1979; Zellweger, Pavone, Biondi, Cimino, Gulotta, Hart, Ionescu, Mollica, and Schicken, 1980).

Total loss-of-function is of course also expected with shifts of the reading frame resulting in an early termination of the protein. This is exemplified by two human mutations associated with Becker myotonia (Meyer-Kleine et al., 1994; Heine et al., 1994), and also with defects in splicing as with the transposon insertion in ADR mice (Steinmeyer et al., 1991*b*) and probably with a human point mutation (Lorenz et al., 1994). More subtle mutations should be analyzed functionally. The R496S mutation, which affects a highly conserved arginine in putative transmembrane span D10, was therefore introduced by site-directed mutagenesis into the functional human ClC-1 cDNA. Expression in *Xenopus* oocytes revealed that it indeed leads to a non-functional channel, and coexpression with wild-type (WT) ClC-1 was fully compatible with the associated recessive pattern of inheritance (Lorenz et al., 1994).

The fact that total loss-of-function of the gene product of one allele results in recessive disease implies that the dominant mutations found in Thomsen's disease must interfere with the functional expression from the normal allele. This dominant negative effect is most easily explained with a (homo)multimeric channel complex. In such a model, one would postulate that the mutated channel protein does not yield functional channels in a homomultimeric complex; moreover, it should still be able to associate with wild-type channel subunits encoded by the normal allele, yielding again nonfunctional channels. Thereby, mutated subunits suppress the function of the normal allele, leading to a dominant negative phenotype.

If one assumes that a single mutated subunit is able to completely abolish channel activity in a multimeric complex with WT subunits, the dominant negative effect will be stronger with a larger number of subunits. With a dimeric channel, 25% of channels will be functional (wild-type; WT) when equal amounts of mutated and WT subunits are present; with a tetrameric channel, in contrast, only 6% of the channels will be functional (Fig. 2). Thus, currents measured in experiments in which different ratios of WT and mutant subunits are coexpressed should give us information on the stoichiometry of the channel complex.

Both the original Thomsen mutation P480L (Steinmeyer et al., 1994) as well as a mutation (G230E) found in a Canadian family with dominant myotonia congenita (George et al., 1993) were inserted into the human ClC-1 cDNA. Channels were nonfunctional with either mutation. Surprisingly, coexpression experiments yielded results which seemed at first conflicting: analysis of the P480L mutant suggested that ClC-1 functions as a homotetramer, whereas the data obtained with the G230E mutant were compatible at most with a dimer (Steinmeyer et al., 1994). This apparent contradiction could be resolved with the observation that coexpression of mutant G230E and WT channels yielded functional, though slightly altered channels at a low mutant/WT concentration ratio. While the WT channel is blocked by iodide in the positive voltage range (where iodide is driven into the channel), this block is

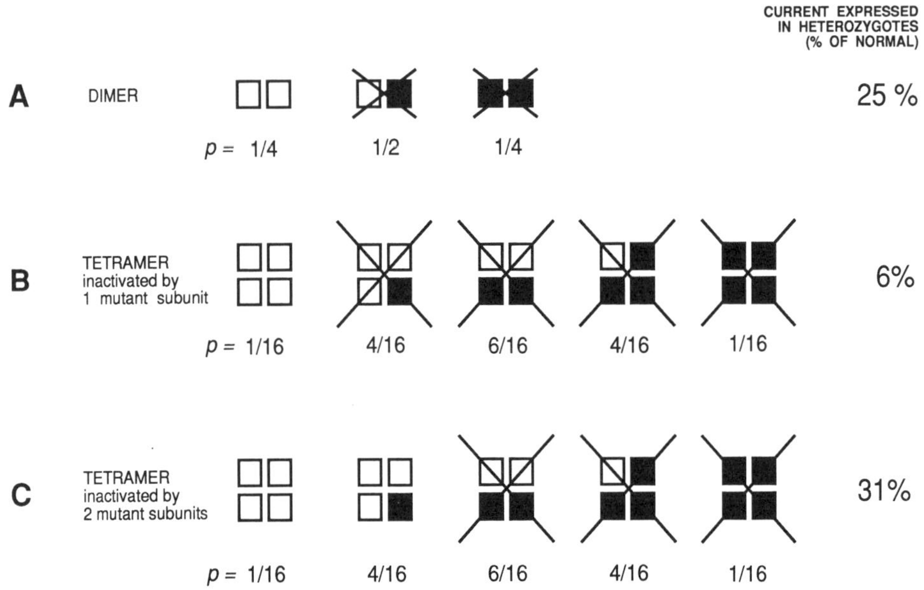

Figure 2. Models to explain negative dominant effects in terms of a multimeric channel model. The channel is either assumed to be a homodimer (*A*) or a homotetramer (*B* and *C*). If one mutated subunit in a multimeric complex is sufficient to abolish channel activity, and if both subunits are present in equal concentrations as probably in a heterozygote, macroscopic current will be reduced to 25% for a dimeric channel (*A*) or to 6% in a tetrameric channel (*B*). If the tetramer tolerates the insertion of one mutant subunit, but not of two, 31% of current is predicted (*C*). The experiments in Steinmeyer et al. (1994) provide evidence for a (homo)tetrameric channel; the "original" Thomsen mutation P480L behaves as in scheme (*B*), while the partially dominant mutation G230E (George et al., 1993) leads to functional channels with altered properties when just one mutant copy is inserted (Steinmeyer et al., 1994).

very much reduced upon coexpression with G230E. This provided us with a rather specific blocker for WT ClC-1 (Steinmeyer et al., 1994). ClC-1 currents measured in the presence of the blocker iodide increased steeply upon the addition of small amounts of mutant (G230E) cRNA to the expression system, showing that functional, iodide-resistant heteromultimeric channels were formed. Increasing the amount of mutated cRNA further led then to a decrease of currents, compatible with the dominant nature of this mutation. This is convincing and independent evidence that ClC-1 must have at least three subunits: a minimum of two subunits is necessary to explain the formation of channels with altered properties, whereas a third one is needed to account for the reduction of currents at higher mutant concentration. Thus, we proposed (Steinmeyer et al., 1994) a model in which the incorporation of one mutated subunit into a tetrameric channel complex produced channels with slightly altered properties. Incorporation of two or more mutated subunits destroys channel function altogether (Fig. 2). In a heterozygote expressing equal amounts of mutated and WT proteins, this will result in a reduction of total current to ~30%. This is fully compatible with experiments titrating the G230E mutant, and fully agrees with the titration experiments using the more dominant P480L mutant of Dr. Thomsen which directly indicated a tetrameric channel.

Thus, this mechanism provides an easy explanation for the fact that some mutations in ClC-1 are dominant and others recessive. Analysis of the G230E mutant also demonstrates that the border between dominant and recessive mutations may be blurred, as the reduction of ClC-1 currents predicted for a heterozygote (≈30%) is close to the limit where myotonic symptoms become apparent. Our functional analysis of the G230E mutant in *Xenopus* oocytes was recently supported nicely by the genetic and clinical analysis of an American family with myotonia which at first seemed to be recessive (E. Hoffman, personal communication). Genetic analysis indicated the presence of the G230E mutation. This suggests that this mutation can have a decreased penetrance, possibly depending on the genetic background. Thus, at this point in time, only the original Thomsen mutation (P480L) may qualify as a fully dominant Thomsen-type mutation.

A multimeric structure of ClC-1, as indicated by these (partially) dominant mutations, also fits nicely with other observations. The *Torpedo* channel ClC-0 (Jentsch et al., 1990) has been proposed to be double barreled, having two independent, identical pores (Miller and White, 1984; Bauer et al., 1991). In the absence of an internal repeat structure in the protein this strongly suggests at least a dimer. While our results suggest a tetramer for ClC-1 (Steinmeyer et al., 1994), sucrose density centrifugation of ClC-0 rather suggests a dimer (Middleton et al., 1994). At present, the reason for this discrepancy is unclear.

As described above, several predicted truncations of the protein (as in the ADR mouse [Steinmeyer et al., 1991*b*], or with deletions leading to shifts in reading frames [Meyer-Kleine et al., 1994; Heine et al., 1994]) result in recessive mutations. Assuming that our model of the multimeric structure of the channel is correct, this could mean that either these truncated subunits can no longer associate with the normal ones (which would otherwise be inactivated), or that the corresponding mRNA or the truncated protein is unstable. These results are in contrast to the properties of the truncated *Shaker* potassium channel, which exerts a dominant negative phenotype in transgenic *Drosophila* (Gisselmann, Sewing, Madsen, Mallart, Angaut-Petit, Muller-Holtkamp, Ferrús, and Pongs, 1989).

Thus, the cloning of the skeletal muscle chloride channel ClC-1 (Steinmeyer et al., 1991*a*) has led, within a short period of time, to the demonstration that mutations in this gene can cause both recessive and dominant forms of myotonia. Moreover, careful analysis of mutations causing myotonia has already yielded important results concerning the structure and function of that channel, and, in extension, of that channel family.

Acknowledgements

Work in our laboratory is supported, in part, by the Bundesministerium für Forschung und Technologie, the Deutsche Forschungsgemeinschaft, the Fonds der Chemischen Industrie, and the United States Muscular Dystrophy Association.

References

Abdalla, J., W. L. Casley, H. K. Cousin, A. J. Hudson, E. G. Murphy, F. C. Cornélis, L. Hashimoto, and G. C. Ebers. 1992. Linkage of Thomsen disease to the T-cell-receptor beta (TCRB) locus on chromosome 7q35. *American Journal of Human Genetics.* 51:579–584.

Adachi, M., R. Watanabe-Fukunaga, and S. Nagata. 1993. Aberrant transcription caused by the insertion of an early transposable element in an intron of the Fas antigen gene of *lpr* mice. *Proceedings of the National Academy of Sciences, USA.* 90:1756–1760.

Adrian, R. H., and S. H. Bryant. 1974. On the repetitive discharge in myotonic muscle fibres. *Journal of Physiology.* 240:505–515.

Bauer, C. K., K. Steinmeyer, J. R. Schwarz, and T. J. Jentsch. 1991. Completely functional double-barreled chloride channel expressed from a single *Torpedo* cDNA. *Proceedings of the National Academy of Sciences, USA.* 88:11052–11056.

Becker, P. E. 1977. Myotonia Congenita and Syndromes Associated with Myotonia. Thieme, Stuttgart.

Becker, P. E. 1979. Heterozygote manifestation in recessive generalized myotonia. *Human Genetics.* 46:325–329.

Brook, J. D., M. E. McCurrach, H. G. Harley, A. J. Buckler, D. Church, H. Aburatani, K. Hunter, V. P. Stanton, J.-P. Thirion, T. Hudson, R. Sohn, B. Zemelman, R. G. Snell, S. A. Rundle, S. Crow, J. Davies, P. Shelbourne, J. Buxton, C. Jones, V. Juvonen, K. Johnson, P. S. Harper, D. J. Shaw, and D. E. Housman. 1992. Molecular basis of myotonic dystrophy: expansion of a trinucleotide (CTG) repeat at the 3′ end of a transcript encoding a protein kinase family member. *Cell.* 68:799–808.

Bryant, S. H., and A. Morales-Aguilera. 1971. Chloride conductance in normal and myotonic muscle fibres and the action of monocarboxylic aromatic acids. *Journal of Physiology.* 219:367–383.

Camerino, D., and S. H. Bryant. 1976. Effects of denervation and colchicine treatment on the chloride conductance of rat skeletal muscle fibers. *Journal of Neurobiology.* 7:221–228.

Conte Camerino, D., A. De Luca, M. Mambrini, and G. Vrbovà. 1989. Membrane ionic conductances in normal and denervated skeletal muscle of the rat during development. *Pflügers Archiv.* 413:568–570.

Fontaine, B., T. S. Khurana, E. P. Hoffman, G. A. P. Bruns, J. L. Haines, J. A. Trofatter, M. P. Hanson, J. Rich, H. McFarlane, D. M. Yasek, D. Romano, J. F. Gusella, and R. H. Brown, Jr. 1990. Hyperkalemic periodic paralysis and the adult muscle sodium channel α-subunit gene. *Science.* 250:1000–1002.

Franke, C., P. A. Iaizzo, H. Hatt, W. Spittelmeister, K. Ricker, and F. Lehmann-Horn. 1991. Altered Na^+ channel activity and reduced Cl^- conductance cause hyperexcitability in recessive generalized myotonia (Becker). *Muscle Nerve.* 14:762–770.

Fu, Y.-H., A. Pizzuti, R. G. Fenwick, Jr., J. King, S. Rajnarayan, P. W. Dunne, J. Dubel, G. A. Nasser, T. Ashizawa, P. de Jong, B. Wieringa, R. Korneluk, M. B. Perryman, H. F. Epstein, and C. T. Caskey. 1992. An unstable triplet repeat in a gene related to myotonic muscular dystrophy. *Science.* 255:1256–1258.

George, A. L., M. A. Crackower, J. A. Abdalla, A. J. Hudson, and G. C. Ebers. 1993. Molecular basis of Thomsen's disease (autosomal dominant myotonia congenita). *Nature Genetics.* 3:305–309.

Gisselmann, G., S. Sewing, B. W. Madsen, A. Mallart, D. Angaut-Petit, F. Müller-Holtkamp, A. Ferrús, and O. Pongs. 1989. The interference of truncated with normal potassium channel subunits leads to abnormal behaviour in transgenic *Drosophila melanogaster. EMBO Journal.* 8:2359–2364.

Gronemeier, M., A. Condie, J. Prosser, K. Steinmeyer, T. J. Jentsch, and H. Jockusch. 1994. Nonsense and missense mutations in the muscular chloride channel *Clc-1* of myotonic mice. *Journal of Biological Chemistry.* 269:5963–5967.

Gründer, S., A. Thiemann, M. Pusch, and T. J. Jentsch. 1992. Regions involved in the opening of ClC-2 chloride channel by voltage and cell volume. *Nature.* 360:759–762.

Heine, R., A. L. George, U. Pika, F. Deymeer, R. Rüdel, and F. Lehmann-Horn. 1994. Proof of a nonfunctional muscle chloride channel in recessive myotonia congenita (Becker) by detection of a 4 bp deletion. *Human Molecular Genetics.* 3:1123–1128.

Iaizzo, P. A., C. Franke, H. Hatt, W. Spittelmeister, K. Ricker, R. Rüdel, and F. Lehmann-Horn. 1991. Altered sodium channel behaviour causes myotonia in dominantly inherited myotonia congenita. *Neuromuscular Disorders.* 1:47–53.

Jentsch, T. J., K. Steinmeyer, and G. Schwarz. 1990. Primary structure of *Torpedo marmorata* chloride channel isolated by expression cloning in *Xenopus* oocytes. *Nature.* 348:510–514.

Jentsch, T. J. 1994. Molecular physiology of anion channels. *Current Opinion in Cell Biology.* 6:600–606.

Kieferle, S., P. Fong, M. Bens, A. Vandewalle, and T. J. Jentsch. 1994. Two highly homologous members of the ClC chloride channel family in both rat and human kidney. *Proceedings of the National Academy of Sciences, USA.* 91:6943–6947.

Klocke, R., K. Steinmeyer, T. J. Jentsch, and H. Jockusch. 1994. Role of innervation, excitability, and myogenic factors on the muscular chloride channel ClC-1: a study on normal and myotonic muscle. *Journal of Biological Chemistry.* 269:27635–27639.

Koch, M. C., K. Steinmeyer, C. Lorenz, K. Ricker, F. Wolf, M. Otto, B. Zoll, F. Lehmann-Horn, K. H. Grzeschik, and T. J. Jentsch. 1992. The skeletal muscle chloride channel in dominant and recessive myotonia. *Science.* 257:797–800.

Koch, M. C., K. Ricker, M. Otto, F. Wolf, B. Zoll, C. Lorenz, K. Steinmeyer, and T. J. Jentsch. 1993. Evidence for genetic homogeneity in autosomal recessive generalised myotonia (Becker). *Journal of Medical Genetics.* 30:914–917.

Kwiecinski, H., F. Lehmann-Horn, and R. Rüdel. 1988. Drug-induced myotonia in human intercostal muscle. *Muscle Nerve.* 11:576–581.

Lipicky, R. J., and S. H. Bryant. 1966. Sodium, potassium, and chloride fluxes in intercostal muscle from normal goats and goats with hereditary myotonia. *Journal of General Physiology.* 50:89–111.

Lipicky, R. J., S. H. Bryant, and J. H. Salmon. 1971. Cable parameters, sodium, potassium, chloride, and water content, and potassium efflux in isolated external intercostal muscle of normal volunteers and patients with myotonia congenita. *Journal of Clinical Investigation.* 50:2091–2103.

Lorenz, C., C. Meyer-Kleine, K. Steinmeyer, M. C. Koch, and T. J. Jentsch. 1994. Genomic organization of the human muscle chloride channel ClC-1 and analysis of novel mutations leading to Becker-type myotonia. *Human Molecular Genetics.* 3:941–946.

Mahadevan, M., C. Tsilfidis, L. Sabourin, G. Shutler, C. Amemiya, G. Jansen, C. Neville, M. Narang, J. Barceló, K. O'Hoy, S. Leblond, J. Earle-MacDonald, P. J. de Jong, B. Wieringa, and R. G. Korneluk. 1992. Myotonic dystrophy mutation: an unstable CTG repeat in the 3′ untranslated region of the gene. *Science.* 255:1253–1255.

McClatchey, A. I., P. van den Berg, M. A. Pericak-Vance, W. Raskind, C. Verellen, D. McKenna-Yasek, R. Keshav, J. L. Haines, T. Bird, R. H. Brown Jr., and J. F. Gusella. 1992. Temperature-sensitive mutations in the III–IV cytoplasmic loop region of the skeletal muscle sodium channel gene in paramyotonia congenita. *Cell.* 68:769–774.

Mehrke, G., H. Brinkmeier, and H. Jockusch. 1988. The myotonic mouse mutant ADR: Electrophysiology of the muscle fiber. *Muscle Nerve.* 11:440–446.

Meyer-Kleine, C., K. Ricker, M. Otto, and M. C. Koch. 1994. A recurrent 14 bp deletion in the CLCN1 gene associated with generalized myotonia (Becker). *Human Molecular Genetics.* 3:1015–1016.

Middleton, R. E., D. J. Pheasant, and C. Miller. 1994. Purification, reconstitution and subunit composition of a voltage-gated chloride channel from *Torpedo* electroplax. *Biochemistry.* 33:13189–13198.

Miller, C., and M. M. White. 1984. Dimeric structure of single chloride channels from *Torpedo* electroplax. *Proceedings of the National Academy of Sciences, USA.* 81:2772–2775.

Palade, P. T., and R. L. Barchi. 1977. Characteristics of the chloride conductance in muscle fibres of rat diaphragm. *Journal of General Physiology.* 69:325–342.

Pusch, M., K. Steinmeyer, and T. J. Jentsch. 1994. Low single-channel conductance of the major skeletal muscle chloride channel, ClC-1. *Biophysical Journal.* 66:149–152.

Reininghaus, J., E. M. Füchtbauer, K. Bertram, and H. Jockusch. 1988. The myotonic mouse mutant ADR: Physiological and histochemical properties of muscle. *Muscle Nerve.* 11:433–439.

Rojas, C. V., J. Wang, L. S. Schwartz, E. P. Hoffman, B. R. Powell, and R. H. Brown, Jr. 1991. A met-to-val mutation in the skeletal muscle Na^+ channel α-subunit in hyperkalaemic period paralysis. *Nature.* 354:387–389.

Rüdel, R., and F. Lehmann-Horn. 1985. Membrane changes in cells from myotonia patients. *Physiological Reviews.* 65:310–356.

Rüdel, R., K. Ricker, and F. Lehmann-Horn. 1988. Transient weakness and altered membrane characteristic in recessive generalized myotonia (Becker). *Muscle Nerve.* 11:202–211.

Steinmeyer, K., C. Ortland, and T. J. Jentsch. 1991*a.* Primary structure and functional expression of a developmentally regulated skeletal muscle chloride channel. *Nature.* 354:301–304.

Steinmeyer, K., R. Klocke, C. Ortland, M. Gronemeier, H. Jockusch, S. Gründer, and T. J. Jentsch. 1991*b.* Inactivation of muscle chloride channel by transposon insertion in myotonic mice. *Nature.* 354:304–308.

Steinmeyer, K., C. Lorenz, M. Pusch, M. C. Koch, and T. J. Jentsch. 1994. Multimeric structure of ClC-1 chloride channel revealed by mutations in dominant myotonia congenita (Thomsen). *EMBO Journal.* 13:737–743.

Thiemann, A., S. Gründer, M. Pusch, and T. J. Jentsch. 1992. A chloride channel widely expressed in epithelial and nonepithelial cells. *Nature.* 356:57–60.

Thomsen, J. 1876. Tonische Krämpfe in willkürlich beweglichen Muskeln in Folge von ererbter psychischer Disposition. *Archiv für Psychiatrie und Nervenkrankheiten.* 6:702–718.

Wischmeyer, E., E. Nolte, R. Klocke, H. Jockusch, and H. Brinkmeier. 1993. Development of electrical myotonia in the ADR mouse: role of chloride conductance in myotubes and neonatal animals. *Neuromuscular Disorders.* 3:267–274.

Zellweger, H., L. Pavone, A. Biondi, V. Cimino, F. Gulotta, M. Hart, V. Ionescu, F. Mollica, and R. Schieken. 1980. Autosomal recessive generalized myotonia. *Muscle Nerve.* 3:176–180.

Chapter 6

Linkage Analysis

Correlating Ion Channels with Disease Using Genetic Linkage Analysis

Garry R. Cutting

Department of Pediatrics and Medicine, The Johns Hopkins University School of Medicine, Center for Medical Genetics, Baltimore, Maryland 21287

Introduction

A critical initial step in associating a channel gene with disease phenotype is to map the location of the gene in the human and murine genomes. Because a number of disease phenotypes have been previously mapped in both species, it is possible that the location of a channel gene may coincide with a previously identified disease locus. If this is the case, then polymorphic DNA markers from the gene can be developed and to determine whether an allele of the candidate gene cosegregates with the disease phenotype. A complete association between the polymorphic marker and the disease phenotype would be highly suggestive that alterations in the gene are responsible for the disease. In this case, the next step would be to identify mutations in the candidate gene in affected individuals.

If the channel gene is not coincident with a previously mapped disease, a survey of reasonable phenotypes can be undertaken. The inheritance pattern of polymorphic markers from the candidate channel gene can be assessed in affected families. Cosegregation of a polymorphic marker with the disease phenotype would suggest that they are linked. In this case a search for mutations can then be undertaken. The evidence of very tight linkage (e.g., no recombinations between the marker and the disease phenotype) in certain pedigrees would suggest that the mutations in the candidate gene may be responsible for the disease. Lack of linkage in other families would suggest either of two situations: (*a*) the linkage observed in other pedigrees occurred by chance or (*b*) genetic heterogeneity exists. In the latter case, mutations in the candidate gene may be responsible for some, but not all cases of a disease.

Mapping a Cloned Gene

Numerous techniques are available for the mapping of cloned genes (McKusick, 1991, 1994). Several of the more commonly used methods will be reviewed briefly. Somatic cell hybrid panels consisting of rodent cell lines containing one or a few human chromosomes are widely used for mapping human genes. DNA is available from multiple hybrid cell panels that include the entire human genome (Creagan and Ruddle, 1977). Amplification of DNA from each of these hybrids using PCR and primers from a single copy region of the candidate gene (e.g., 3′ translated region) is then performed (Cutting, Curristin, Zoghbi, Seldin, and Uhl, 1992). The chromosome content of cell lines that amplifies a product of the appropriate size are compared to obtain a chromosomal assignment. Sublocalization to a specific region of a chromosome can be undertaken using rodent hybrid panels that contains portions of the specific chromosome.

DNA fragments from the channel gene can be used as probes to directly hybridize to metaphase chromosome spreads (Trask, 1991). Direct visualization of a signal from the probe can identify the specific chromosomal location of the channel gene. This can be achieved using the entire cDNA or a genomic DNA fragment from the gene ranging in size from ten thousand to several hundred thousand basepairs. This service is available in many academic centers as well as from numerous commercial laboratories. A third method commonly employed is to perform a linkage study in families or individuals which have previously been studied with DNA markers covering the entire genome (White, Leppert, Bishop, Barker, Berkowitz, Brown, Callahan, Holm, and Jerominski, 1985). Mapping in humans is most easily facilitated by the availability of a reference panel of families from the Centre d'Etude du Polymorphisme Humain (CEPH) in Paris (Atwood et al., 1994). Cosegregation of a polymorphic marker from the gene of interest and previously mapped polymorphic markers establishes the map location. Similar studies can be performed in mice using interspecific backcrossing (Cutting et al., 1992; Watson, D'Eustachio, Mock, Steinberg, Morse, Oakey, Howard, Rochelle, and Seldin, 1992). In this case, the investigator takes advantage of polymorphic variants that differ between the two species of mice. A fourth technique uses yeast artificial chromosomes (YACs). As part of the Human Genome Project, YACs covering entire regions of human chromosomes have been assembled and catalogued (Bellanne-Chantelot, Lacroix, Ougen, Bellauet, Beaufels, Bertrand, Georges, Gilbert, Gros, and Lucotte, 1992). Individual YACs that are individually sorted into large arrays that can be PCR amplified to determine which YACs contain the gene of interest. Because the YACs have been previously localized, this method provides an immediate map location as well as flanking genomic DNA.

Determining Whether a Phenotype Colocalizes with a Cloned Gene

After mapping of the gene to a particular location in the human or murine genome, the second step is to determine whether it colocalizes with a previously mapped phenotype. There are two computerized databases that are useful for this purpose, the Genome Database (GDB) and the Online Mendelian Inheritance in Man (OMIM). OMIM has been an ongoing project of Dr. Victor McKusick to catalogue all of the reported disorders with evidence of X-linked, autosomal dominant or autosomal recessive inheritance and is also available in hardcopy as Mendelian Inheritance in Man (McKusick, 1994). These databases are integrated to cross-reference inherited diseases with map locations and DNA polymorphisms from these map locations.

There are two other important sources. Human chromosome mapping workshops are held yearly to determine the locations of newly mapped genes and disease loci upon each human chromosome. Editors are assigned to each human chromosome and yearly reports on the most recent mapping data are published in journals such as *Genomics* or *Cytogenetics* and *Cell Genetics* (Green, 1992). Resources important for the mapping of murine traits are available in publications from the Jackson Laboratory in Bar Harbor, Maine (Davisson, 1994; Sharp and Davisson, 1994; Nadeau, Davisson, Doolittle, Grant, Hillyard, Krowsky, and Roderick, 1992).

Linkage Analysis

The primary goal of linkage analysis is to determine if a polymorphism from a candidate gene segregates with the disease phenotype. The strength of linkage depends upon the number of individuals studied with unambiguous results. This approach is particularly powerful when analyzing individuals and families whose disease has been linked to a specific chromosomal locus. In this situation, genetic heterogeneity has been eliminated, therefore, a recombination between a polymorphic DNA marker from the channel gene and the disease locus indicates that the two may be physically close but not associated with the disease locus (Fig. 1). Recombinations are identified by comparing the inheritance pattern of the channel gene polymorphisms with the disease phenotype.

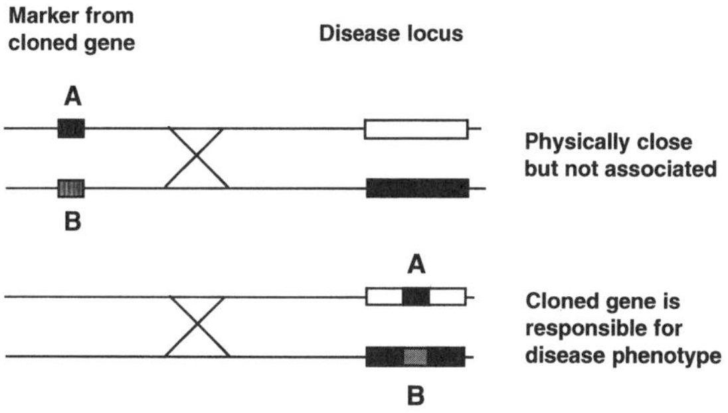

Figure 1. Diagram showing how recombinations can help determine whether a DNA marker colocalizes with a disease locus. Each line represents a chromosome with an X indicating the location of a recombination event. (*Open rectangle*) Normal gene. (*Filled rectangle*) Mutated gene.

The initial step in linkage analysis is the development of polymorphic markers. DNA polymorphism is a condition in which one of two different but normal nucleotide sequences can exist at a particular site in DNA. For a locus to be considered polymorphic, the less frequent sequence must have a frequency of 1% or higher in the population. Restriction-site polymorphism is a specific type of DNA polymorphism in which the sequence of one form of the polymorphism contains a recognition sequence for a particular endonuclease and the sequence of the other form lacks such a recognition sequence. These polymorphisms must be stable and inherited in an Mendelian codominant fashion. The more frequent that a polymorphism is found in the heterozygous state the more useful the polymorphism because genes can be distinguished from each other and their inheritance patterns can be monitored. The second type of polymorphism, called a variable number of tandem repeats (VNTR), capitalizes on the availability of repeat sequences in the human genome which are highly variable. At a particular locus, the repeats vary in length to produce a large number of different alleles. This considerably enhances the possibility that an individual would be heterozygous at this locus. Both types of polymorphism can be detected easily using the polymerase chain reaction. Primers are chosen to amplify the polymorphic site and flanking DNA. A restriction-site polymor-

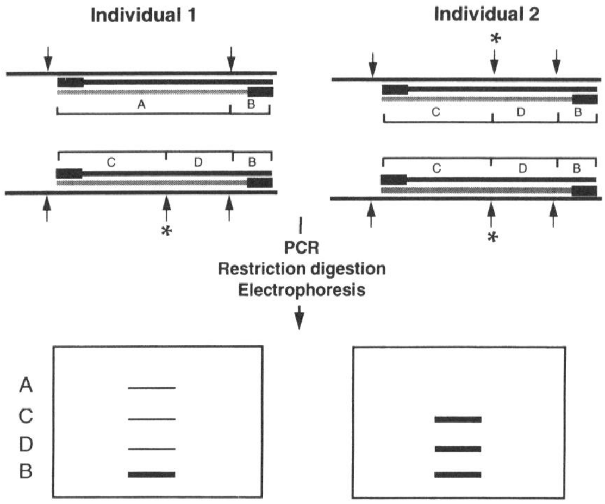

Figure 2. Detection of a restriction-site polymorphism by PCR. (*Arrows*) Sites digested by a restriction enzyme with the asterisk marking a polymorphic site. (*A–D*) DNA fragments expected after digestion of the PCR product. Individual 1 is heterozygous for the polymorphic site as shown by the presence of fragments *A, C,* and *D.* Fragment *B* is always present and serves as a control for enzymatic digestion. Individual 2 is homozygous for the presence of the polymorphic site and has fragments *C* and *D* only.

phism is detected by enzyme digestion whereas VNTR alleles are determined on the basis of the size of amplified products (Figs. 2 and 3).

Pedigrees segregating a disease that colocalizes with the candidate gene can be analyzed with the polymorphic markers. An example of typing two pedigress with a diallelic polymorphism is shown in Fig. 4. In this situation, the autosomal recessive disorder in both families has been previously mapped using anonymous DNA markers. This locus coincides with the map location of the channel gene. The parents are heterozygous for polymorphisms from each candidate gene, therefore, their two genes can be differentiated. On the left, the three affected individuals received the B variant from each parent. None of the unaffected children have the same genotype as the affected children (BB) suggesting linkage between the B allele of the candidate gene and the disease phenotype. The family on the right has two affected children with the AA genotype suggesting linkage between the A polymorphism of the channel gene and the disease gene. However, the third affected child inherited A and B polymorphisms indicating a recombination has occurred between the channel gene

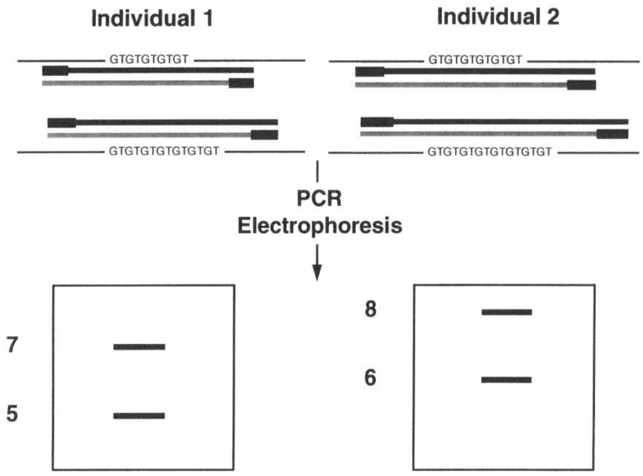

Figure 3. Detection of a VNTR polymorphism by PCR. DNA fragments of slightly different length are amplified from the polymorphic (GT) repeat. Individuals 1 and 2 are heterozygous for repeats of 5 and 7, and 6 and 8, respectively.

marker and the disease phenotype. This recombination indicates that the channel gene and disease gene, although mapping to the same location in the genome, are not one and the same.

Linkage Studies of Unmapped Disease Phenotypes

In situations where a channel gene does not coincide with a previously mapped disease, it is then possible to survey carefully selected inherited diseases that may be caused by defects in the ion channel. This is a four step process: (*a*) disease selection; (*b*) collection of families; (*c*) development of polymorphic markers; and (*d*) linkage analysis. The first step is the identification of diseases with symptoms that match the predicted consequences of channel gene dysfunction. This approach has been successfully used for skeletal muscle myotonias where tissues from the affected individuals were known to have a defect in either sodium or chloride conduction (Ptacek, George, Barchi, Griggs, Riggs, Robertson, and Leppert, 1992; Rojas, Wang, Schwartz, Hoffman, Powell, and Brown, 1991; Koch, Steinmeyer, Lorenz, Ricker, Wolf, Otto, Zoll, Lehmann-Horn, Grzeschik, and Jentsch, 1992). Two criteria that may be helpful but not essential during phenotype selection are: (*a*) the pattern of expression of the channel gene matches the organs and/or tissues affected in the

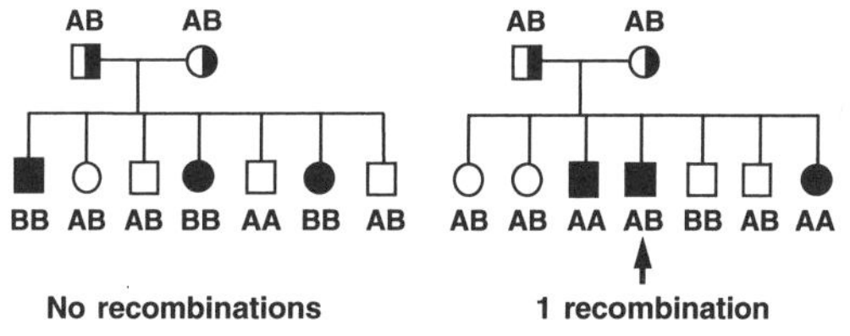

Figure 4. Testing of two families segregating an autosomal recessive disease that maps to the same location as a channel gene. The results of typing all individuals with a DNA marker from the channel gene with polymorphism *A* and *B* are shown. Parents in both families are heterozygous (*AB*). (*Filled circles or squares*) Homozygous affected individuals. (*Half-filled symbols*) Obligate heterozygotes.

disorder; (*b*) the mode of inheritance is compatible with the understanding of the protein function. In the latter case, a defective channel that normally functions as part of a multimeric complex would be expected to cause a dominant disorder. However there are exceptions, notably in chloride channel myotonias caused by defects in the voltage-gated chloride channel-1 (CIC-1) that display both autosomal dominant and autosomal recessive inheritance (Koch et al., 1992).

In the second step, DNA samples from families have to be collected to facilitate linkage studies. Precise diagnosis is essential to avoid erroneous identification of a recombination. Large multigenerational families are most helpful for autosomal dominant and X-linked traits. In recessive disorders, linkage studies require the use of many families with two or more affected siblings. The development of stable polymorphisms which have a high degree of heterozygosity has been discussed previously. The final step is linkage analysis and the value of informative markers is evident during the phase. Shown in Fig. 5 is a linkage study of an autosomal dominant phenotype in an extended pedigree with five affected individuals. The maternal grandfather (generation I, *filled square*) is informative because his two genes can be differentiated (*A* or *B*). Linkage of the B polymorphism with the disease is suggested by the following. In the generation II, the male with genotype AA is unaffected while both of his affected sisters inherited a B from their affected father. However, in the next generation, one of the affected daughters has married a man who is heterozygous AB. Therefore, it is not possible to determine unambigously whether the B polymorphism is linked to the disease locus. For example, one affected child in generation III carries the genotype BB suggesting that B is linked to the disease. The affected male in this sibship however has genotype AB and it cannot be determined whether he inherited the B polymorphism from his father or from his mother. In this case, the family is partially informative and the inheritance pattern is consistent with linkage. This pattern of inheritance could have occurred by chance alone. Similar results from a number of families will increase the likelihood that this channel gene is linked to the disease.

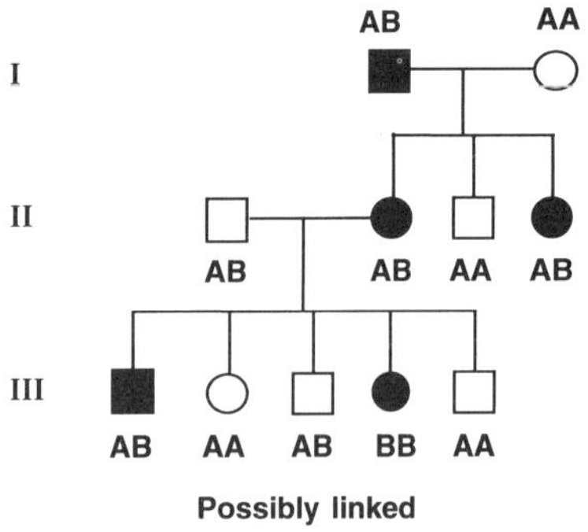

Figure 5. Linkage analysis of three generation family segregating an autosomal dominant condition using a diallelic polymorphism from a candidate channel gene. (*Filled symbols*) Affected individuals. Each generation is denoted by a roman numeral.

The probability of a statistically significant association between a disease and a channel gene can be assessed by calculating a logarithm of the odds of linkage (LOD) score (Ott, 1991). If few recombinations occur per meiosis then the LOD score will be high. If a large number of recombinations per informative meiosis are observed then the LOD score is low. A polymorphic marker with an LOD score > 3 indicates chances of linkage are 1,000 to 1 over the chances of nonlinkage which has generally been viewed as "proof of linkage." However, the investigator should keep in mind that this is a statistical representation of the possibility of linkage (Risch, 1991). When an LOD > 3 has been obtained, mutation analysis of the linked gene is usually undertaken. The discovery of a deleterious mutation in a candidate gene in an affected individual generally proves the association between a gene and a disease. Depending on the size of the gene, the identification of a deleterious mutation can be a difficult task. Four commonly employed techniques are their detection rate, advantages and disadvantages are illustrated in Table I.

Identification of Deleterious Mutations

Mutations that introduce premature termination signals such as nonsense, frameshift, or splicing alterations are usually deleterious. However, mutations that are predicted to alter splicing and those causing an amino acid substitution (missense mutation) may or may not be deleterious. In the latter case, there are several criteria one can use to differentiate between deleterious and neutral missense mutations. The "gold" standard is to determine whether an alteration changes the function of the expressed protein. In some cases, this may not be feasible. Therefore, circumstantial evidence can be used. The observation of a de novo mutation in sporadic cases of the disease provides excellent evidence that a mutation is associated with disease. Absence of an alteration in a selected sample of the normal population decreases the possibility that the change may be a neutral polymorphism. Considering that protein polymorphism was originally defined as a variation that occurs in 1% or more of the

TABLE I
Comparison of Methods for the Detection of Novel Mutations

Methods	Detection rate	Advantage	Disadvantage
DNA sequencing	100%	Direct analysis	Technical, labor intensive
Single-strand conformation polymorphism	~80%	Simple	Short fragments, radioactivity
Denaturing gradient gel electrophoresis	100%	Nonradioactive, heteroduplex pattern	GC clamped primers, computer modeling
Chemical cleavage of mismatch	100%	Large fragments, location	Toxic chemical, several steps
Enzymatic cleavage of mismatch	70%	Large fragments, location	Low sensitivity, RNA synthesis

population, investigators usually analyze at least 100 normal genes to exclude polymorphism. Alteration of a highly conservative amino acid or discovery of multiple mutations in the same amino acid also provides evidence that an alteration is deleterious. Optimally, conservation should be present across evolutionary distant species or members of a superfamily of genes. The nature of the amino acid change can be suggestive such as alteration in the charge of the residue. Changes of this type have been shown to be normal variants, for example, the glycine to glutamic acid mutation observed in the voltage-gated chloride channel 1 (Steinmeyer, Lorenz, Pusch, Koch, and Jentsch, 1994). Finally, linkage of a mutation with the disease has been used to demonstrate that an alteration is deleterious. This can be misleading because neutral mutations, like deleterious mutations, can show linkage to a disease phenotype.

References

Attwood, J., M. Chiano, A. Collins, H. Donis-Keller, N. Dracopoli, J. Fountain, C. Falk, D. Goudie, J. Gusella, J. Haines, J. A. L. Armour, A. J. Jeffreys, D. Kweatkowski, M. Lathrop, T. Matise, H. Northrup, M. A. Pericak-Yance, J. Phillips, A. Retief, E. Robson, D. Shields, S. Slaugenhaupt, G. Vergnaud, J. Weber, J. Weissenbach, R. White, J. Yates, and S. Poney. 1994. CEPH consortium map of chromosome 9. *Genomics.* 19:203–214.

Bellanne-Chantelot, C., B. Lacroix, P. Ougen, A. Bellauet, S. Beaufels, S. Bertrand, I. Georges, F. Gilbert, I. Gros, and G. Lucotte. 1992. Mapping the whole human genome by fingerprinting yeast artificial chromosomes. *Cell.* 70:1059–1068.

Creagan, R. P., and F. H. Ruddle. 1977. New approaches to human gene mapping by somatic cell genetics. *In* Molecular Structure of Human Chromosomes. J. J. Yunis, editor. Academic Press, New York. 89–142.

Cutting, G. R., S. Curristin, H. Zoghbi, B. O'Hara, M. F. Seldin, and G. R. Uhl. 1992. Identification of a putative gamma-aminobutyric acid (GABA) receptor subunit rho_2 cDNA and colocalization of the genes encoding rho_2 (GABRR2) and rho(GABRR1) to human chromosome 6q14-q21 and mouse chromosome 4. *Genomics.* 12:801–806.

Davisson, M. T. 1990. The Jackson Laboratory mouse mutant resource. *Laboratory Animals.* 19:23–29.

Green, P. 1992. Genetic analysis workshop 7: mapping chromosome 21 linkage markers. *Cytogenetics and Cell Genetics.* 59:77–79.

Koch, M. C., K. Steinmeyer, C. Lorenz, K. Ricker, F. Wolf, M. Otto, B. Zoll, F. Lehmann-Horn, K. Grzeschik, T. J. Jentsch. 1992. The skeletal muscle chloride channel in dominant and recessive human myotonia. *Science.* 257:797–800.

McKusick, V. A. 1991. Current trends in mapping human genes. *FASEB Journal.* 5:12–20.

McKusick, V. A. 1994. Mendelian Inheritance in Man. Johns Hopkins University Press. Baltimore, MD. 3009 pp.

Nadeau, J. H., M. T. Davisson, D. P. Doolittle, P. Grant, A. L. Hillyard, M. R. Kosowsky, and T. H. Roderick. 1992. Comparative map for mice and humans. *Mammalian Genome.* 3:480–536.

Ott, J. 1991. Analysis of Human Genetic Linkage. Johns Hopkins University Press. Baltimore, MD. 328 pp.

Ptacek, L. J., A. L. George, Jr., R. L. Barchi, R. C. Griggs, J. E. Riggs, M. Robertson, and M. F. Leppert. 1992. Mutations in an S4 segment of the adult skeletal muscle sodium channel cause paramyotonia congenita. *Neuron.* 8:891–897.

Risch, N. 1991. Genetic linkage: interpreting lod scores. *Science.* 25:803–804.

Rojas, C. V., J. Wang, L. S. Schwartz, E. P. Hoffman, B. R. Powell, and R. H. Brown, Jr. 1991. A Met-to-Val mutation in the skeletal muscle Na^+ channel alpha-subunit in hyperkalaemic periodic paralysis. *Nature.* 254:387–390.

Sharp, J. J., and M. T. Davisson. 1994. The Jackson Laboratory induced mutant resource. *Laboratory Animals.* 23:32–40.

Steinmeyer, K., C. Lorenz, M. Pusch, M. C. Koch, and T. J. Jentsch. 1994. Multimeric structure of ClC-1 chloride channel revealed by mutations in dominant myotonia congenita (Thomsen). *EMBO Journal.* 13:737–743.

Trask, B. J. 1991. Fluorescence *in situ* hybridization: applications in cytogenetics and gene mapping. *Trends in Genetics.* 7:149–151.

Watson, M. L., P. D'Eustachio, B. A. Mock, A. D. Steinberg, H. C. Morse, III, R. J. Oakey, T. A. Howard, J. M. Rochelle, and M. F. Seldin. 1992. A linkage map of mouse chromosome 1 using an interspecific cross segregating for the gld autoimmunity mutation. *Mammalian Genome.* 2:158–171.

White, R., M. Leppert, D. T. Bishop, D. Barker, J. Berkowitz, C. Brown, P. Callahan, T. Holm, and L. Jerominski. 1985. Construction of linkage maps with DNA markers for human chromosomes. *Nature.* 313:101–105.

List of Contributors

O. Augustinas, Research Institute, Hospital for Sick Children, Toronto, Ontario M5G 1X8, Canada

Robert L. Barchi, Departments of Neurology and Neuroscience, and the Mahoney Institute of Neurological Sciences, University of Pennsylvania School of Medicine, Philadelphia, Pennsylvania 19104

F. Becq, Department of Physiology, McGill University, Montréal, Québec, Canada H3G 1Y6

Heinrich Brinkmeier, Department of General Physiology, University of Ulm, D-89081 Ulm, Germany

X.-B. Chang, S. C. Johnson Medical Research Center, Mayo Clinic Scottsdale, Scottsdale, Arizona 85259

Nirupa Chaudhari, Department of Physiology, Colorado State University, Fort Collins, Colorado 80523

Garry R. Cutting, Department of Pediatrics and Medicine, The Johns Hopkins University School of Medicine, Center for Medical Genetics, Baltimore, Maryland 21287

Victor Dubowitz, Department of Paediatrics and Neonatal Medicine, Hammersmith Hospital, London, W120NN, United Kingdom

Stewart R. Durell, The Laboratory of Mathematical Biology, DCBDC, National Cancer Institute, National Institutes of Health, Bethesda, Maryland 20892

Bertrand Fontaine, INSERM U134, Fédération de Neurologie, Hôpital de la Salpêtrière, 75013 Paris, France

Barry Ganetzky, Laboratory of Genetics, University of Wisconsin, Madison, Wisconsin 53706

Alfred L. George, Department of Medicine, Vanderbilt University School of Medicine, Nashville, Tennessee 37232

H. Robert Guy, Laboratory of Molecular and Cellular Bioenergetics, Department of Biological Chemistry, The Johns Hopkins University, School of Medicine, Baltimore, Maryland 21205-2185

J. W. Hanrahan, Department of Physiology, McGill University, Montréal, Québec, Canada H3G 1Y6

Roland Heine, Department of Applied Physiology, University of Ulm, D-89081 Ulm, Germany

Eric P. Hoffman, Departments of Molecular Genetics and Biochemistry, Human Genetics, and Pediatrics, University of Pittsburgh, Pittsburgh, Pennsylvania 15261

William F. Hopkins, Geriatric Research, Education, and Clinical Center, Veterans Affairs Medical Center, Seattle, Washington 98108; and Departments of Medicine and Pharmacology, University of Washington School of Medicine, Seattle, Washington 98195

Richard Horn, Department of Physiology, Thomas Jefferson University School of Medicine, Philadelphia, Pennsylvania 19107

T. J. Jensen, S. C. Johnson Medical Research Center, Mayo Clinic Scottsdale, Scottsdale, Arizona 85259

Thomas J. Jentsch, Center for Molecular Neurobiology (ZMNH), Hamburg University, D-20246 Hamburg, Germany

Sen Ji, Departments of Neurology and Neuroscience, and the Mahoney Institute of Neurological Sciences, University of Pennsylvania School of Medicine, Philadelphia, Pennsylvania 19104

Karin Jurkat-Rott, Department of Applied Physiology, University of Ulm, D-89081 Ulm, Germany

Mark T. Keating, Cardiology Division, Department of Human Genetics and the Eccles Program in Human Molecular Biology and Genetics, University of Utah, Salt Lake City, Utah 84112

Young Hee Ko, Laboratory of Molecular and Cellular Bioenergetics, Department of Biological Chemistry, The Johns Hopkins University, School of Medicine, Baltimore, Maryland 21205-2185

Laszlo Kovacs, Department of Physiology, University Medical School of Debrecen, H-4012 Debrecen, Hungary

Frank Lehmann-Horn, Department of Applied Physiology, University of Ulm, D-89081 Ulm, Germany

Claudius Lorenz, Center for Molecular Neurobiology (ZMNH), Hamburg University, D-20246 Hamburg, Germany

David H. MacLennan, Banting and Best Department of Medical Research, University of Toronto, Charles H. Best Institute, Toronto, Ontario, Canada M5G1L6

C. J. Mathews, Department of Physiology, McGill University, Montréal, Québec, Canada H3G 1Y6

Werner Melzer, Department of Applied Physiology, University of Ulm, D-89081 Ulm, Germany

Leo Pallanck, Laboratory of Genetics, University of Wisconsin, Madison, Wisconsin 53706

Peter L. Pedersen, Laboratory of Molecular and Cellular Bioenergetics, Department of Biological Chemistry, The Johns Hopkins University, School of Medicine, Baltimore, Maryland 21205-2185

Michael S. Phillips, Banting and Best Department of Medical Research, University of Toronto, Charles H. Best Institute, Toronto, Ontario, Canada M5G1L6

Louis Ptácek, Department of Neurology, University of Utah, School of Medicine, Salt Lake City, Utah 84132

Michael Pusch, Center for Molecular Neurobiology (ZMNH), Hamburg University, D-20246 Hamburg, Germany

Kenneth Ricker, Department of Applied Physiology, University of Ulm, D-89096 Ulm, Germany

J. R. Riordan, S. C. Johnson Medical Research Center, Mayo Clinic Scottsdale, Scottsdale, Arizona 85259

Gail Robertson, Department of Physiology, University of Wisconsin, Madison, Wisconsin 53706

Ponniah Shenbagamurthi, Laboratory of Molecular and Cellular Bioenergetics, Department of Biological Chemistry, The Johns Hopkins University, School of Medicine, Baltimore, Maryland 21205-2185

Istvan Sipos, Department of Applied Physiology, University of Ulm, D-89081 Ulm, Germany; and Department of Physiology, University Medical School of Debrecen, H-4012 Debrecen, Hungary

Alan E. Smith, Genzyme Corporation, Framingham, Massachusetts 01701

Klaus Steinmeyer, Center for Molecular Neurobiology (ZMNH), Hamburg University, D-20246 Hamburg, Germany

J. A. Tabcharani, Department of Physiology, McGill University, Montréal, Québec, Canada H3G 1Y6

Bruce L. Tempel, Geriatric Research, Education and Clinical Center, Veterans Affairs Medical Center, Seattle, Washington 98108; and Departments of Medicine and Pharmacology, University of Washington School of Medicine, Seattle, Washington 98195

Philip J. Thomas, Department of Physiology, The University of Texas, Southwestern Medical Center at Dallas, Dallas, Texas 75235-9040

Jianzhou Wang, Departments of Molecular Genetics and Biochemistry, Human Genetics, and Pediatrics, University of Pittsburgh School of Medicine, Pittsburgh, Pennsylvania 15261

Jeffrey W. Warmke, Department of Genetics and Molecular Biology, Merck Research Laboratories, Rahway, New Jersey 07065

Subject Index

DATE DUE

GAYLORD 234			PRINTED IN U.S.A.